Child development
Diagnosis and assessment

K. S. Holt MD(USA), MD(Manc.), FRCP, DCH

Emeritus Professor of Developmental Paediatrics,
Institute of Child Health, University of London

Butterworth–Heinemann
London   Boston   Singapore   Sydney   Toronto   Wellington

PART OF REED INTERNATIONAL P.L.C.

First published 1991

© Butterworth–Heinemann Ltd, 1991

British Library Cataloguing in Publication Data

Holt, K. S.
    Child development.
    1. Children. Physical development
    I. Title   II. Holt, K. S. (Kenneth Sunderland).
    Developmental paediatrics
    612.65
    ISBN 0-750-61035-2

Library of Congress Cataloging-in-Publication Data

Holt, K. S. (Kenneth Sunderland)
    Child development: diagnosis and assessment/K.S. Holt.
        p.   cm.
    Based on: Developmental paediatrics. 1977.
    Includes bibliographical references.
    Includes index.
    ISBN 0-750-61035-2
    1. Child development.   I. Holt, K. S. (Kenneth Sunderland).
Developmental paediatrics.   II. Title.
    [DNLM: 1. Child Development.   WS 103 H756c]
    RJ131.H63 1991
    612.6'5–dc20
    DNLM/DLC   90-2684
    for Library of Congress   CIP

Composition by Genesis Typesetting, Laser Quay, Rochester, Kent
Printed and bound by Hartnolls Ltd, Bodmin, Cornwall

Preface

Our children inherit the future. Their best equipment to meet the challenges ahead consists of a healthy body, enquiring mind and stable personality. Prominent amongst those helping children to acquire these vital attributes are paediatricians, i.e. those medical specialists who are concerned with child development and care, and the treatment of children's illnesses.

The above paragraph introduced my book, *Developmental Paediatrics: Perspectives and Practice*, and the statements are as true now as they were in 1977 when that book was published. This present book is based on the earlier one. The contents have been brought up-to-date and rearranged and the title has been changed. I hope that this new book will prove to be as acceptable and useful as the older one.

In recent years there have occurred remarkable increases in understanding of the scientific basis of many disorders, especially in biochemistry, immunology and genetics; and in the range of investigative procedures such as ultrasound and other imaging techniques. Consequently, many paediatricians are preoccupied with these events and are not free to engage in the study and promotion of child development. Nevertheless, this book may serve as a useful reminder and reference for them when they consider the progress of their child patients.

Although not as dramatically as in the case of the scientific specialities, there has also been an increase in interest in child development, and more paediatricians now wish to include developmental work in their practice, so they should find a place for this book in their libraries.

Although an understanding of child development might be considered to be a prerequisite for anyone embarking on a medical career, I have been dismayed to learn how little undergraduates are exposed to the topic. In response to a recent enquiry at medical schools I received comments such as: 'so little time is available to teaching paediatrics,' 'all the other aspects crowd out child development' and 'it is hoped they will learn about child development after qualification'. Hopefully students, either as undergraduates or postgraduates, will find that this publication fills a gap in their knowledge.

In this book I have tried to show the depth and breadth of child development, and to indicate how an understanding of development enriches clinical work, especially work with handicapped children. I hope that reading this book will help paediatricians to appreciate the contributions of other professions such as psychology, therapy and education, and also that members of these other professions who are concerned with the promotion of child health and care will find the book useful and interesting.

In the text the doctor/child is referred to as 'he'. This merely reflects convention and does not represent any bias against the female doctors/children who carry out or are being presented for paediatric examination.

A single-author book has advantages and disadvantages. I am well aware that there are many who could have written sections of this book much better than myself, but with multiple contributors there is a loss of cohesion and continuity. So perhaps readers will accept this contribution as an attempt to show that it is still possible to consider a child as a whole individual and to cover all aspects of child development in practice.

K.S.H.

Acknowledgements

I am only too aware of my reliance upon material from many sources. Throughout this book I have tried to acknowledge the source of all such material, and if there are any omissions, these are due to oversight and not to unawareness of my indebtedness to external assistance.

I am indebted to colleagues, both past and present, and to the many paediatricians who have attended postgraduate courses for their stimulation and support.

The successful preparation of the manuscript was the result of untiring help by Mrs Angela Lovell, and the staff of Butterworths were gently encouraging throughout.

I wish to acknowledge the sources of the following illustrations and tables which are reproduced by permission:

I am indebted to Alison Wisbeach for the line drawing of Figure 7.1 and to Angela Christie for the other line drawings. The latter are based upon tape/slide presentations prepared by myself and the late Dr Mary Sheridan and published by Graves Medical Audiovisual, and by H. F. R. Prechtl and D. J. Beintema (1968) A neurological study of newborn infants, *Clinics Dev. Med.,* **28.** London: Heinemann.

Figure 2.3 from *Gray's Anatomy*, 34th edn, Edinburgh: Churchill Livingstone.

Figure 2.4 from Larroche, J. C. (1966) *Human Development,* Philadelphia: W. B. Saunders Company.

Figure 5.1 from Klaus, M. H., Kennell, J. H., Plumb, N. and Zuelkes, S. (1970) *Pediatrics,* **46**, 187.

Figure 7.2 Murphy, K. P. (1962) *Panorama*, Dec 3, Reading: Linco Acoustics Ltd.

Figure 8.4 based on a poster by Ayerst International.

Figures 13.3 and 13.4 from my book (1965) *Assessment of Cerebral Palsy.* London: Lloyd Luke (Medical Books) Ltd.

Figure 14.1 from Bryant, G. M. (1974) *Developmental Medicine and Child Neurology,* **16**, 475.

Contents

Part I
The basis of development

Chapter 1

Development

Definitions and terminology

Just what do we mean when we speak about child development? *Development* is a process of unfolding, expanding, becoming fuller, more complex and more complete. The term applies to a global impression of the child and encompasses growth, increase in understanding, acquisition of new skills and more sophisticated responses and behaviour.

When studying and evaluating development it is helpful to consider different aspects such as motor development and language development, but then the information has to be put together to provide a fully integrated picture.

To understand development fully, attention has to be given to the underlying mechanisms which make it all possible. Satisfactory development requires a well-formed and normally functioning nervous system; an environment which provides appropriate and adequate nutrition at all stages; opportunities to learn and to act; and both challenges and rewards.

Development is determined by genetic endowment and is modified by biochemical influences and environmental events. Unsatisfactory development arises from poor genetic endowment; deficiencies of essential nutrition, opportunities, challenges and rewards; and the intrusion of damaging and disruptive events. These factors are often cumulative. Thus, individuals with poor genetic endowment are less able than others to provide adequate nutrition and opportunities, and to avoid harmful influences for their families, so that a recurring cycle of disadvantage becomes established. Consequently the differences in health and development of the social classes persist despite increased affluence and attempts to redress the balance (Black, 1980).

Growth is the increase in physical dimensions such as length and weight. The study of growth in childhood is important, but is not dealt with in this text. Normally growth and development proceed together and problems arise when there are discrepancies.

Maturation is a process of ripening and reaching maturity. Although this term is sometimes used synonymously with development, it is usually taken to refer more directly to the basic mechanisms. Thus, in connection with human development, maturation refers to the elaboration of structure and function of the nervous system.

The terms normal and average are used frequently in relation to child development. *Normal* is typical, usual, regular, acceptable, healthy or free of

3

abnormality. *Average* is a calculated point around which other values are dispersed equally.

Both these terms are in everyday use. Confusion arises when they are used loosely and interchangeably. Normal is a descriptive term which can be applied to any child who shows typical characteristics for his age. The term average is derived from statistics and implies that measurements have been taken of some particular feature. A normal child can be in a group with a lot of other normal children. The average child in such a group, with respect to some measured characteristic such as height, weight or intelligence, will have around him other above- and below-average children.

These terms must be used carefully in discussions with parents in order to avoid unnecessary confusion and distress. Parents may describe their child as 'average' when they mean that he appears to them to be normal and typical of their family. Children with widely differing abilities from families in different social classes may be described in this way as 'average'. If parents are told that their child is average intellectually, meaning that his scores on intellectual tests correspond to the 'average' figure for the population, they may think that their child is 'normal and acceptable', when in fact he may be considerably above or below the normal pattern for that particular family.

Unsatisfactory development may take various forms. These are discussed and the terms used are described in later chapters.

Two terms in common use which cause confusion and distress are delay and retardation.

Delay infers that the child's development is not as advanced as it should be and that the rate of development has been slower than what is usually acceptable. Parents often think that a delayed child can be stimulated to catch up or may even do so spontaneously. Catching up requires development at a quicker rate than normal for a period, as illustrated in Figure 1.1.

Retardation is also used when development is below normal expectations. Some resent the term because of the stigma it carries, so it should be used cautiously. Others consider that it means held back and believe that if only the block can be removed the child will progress normally.

Handicapped, disadvantaged, deprived (Sheridan, 1962, 1969)

The unwary may use these terms interchangeably, but they have quite distinct meanings. A *handicapped* child is one who suffers from any continuing disability of body, intellect or personality which is likely to interfere with his normal growth and development or capacity to learn. A *disadvantaged* child is one who suffers from a continuing inadequacy of material, affectional, educational or social provisions, or who is subject to detrimental environmental stresses which are likely to interfere with the growth and development of his body, intellect or personality, and thus prevent him from achieving his inherent potential.

Sheridan made this distinction between handicapped and disadvantaged. The former arises from a disturbance primarily affecting the child, the latter indicates a potentially normal and healthy child whose development is stultified by unfavourable environmental conditions. Although the distinction is a valuable contribution to clear thinking and discussion, it should not be followed too rigidly, because in practice the situations sometimes overlap. Thus, the extent to which a

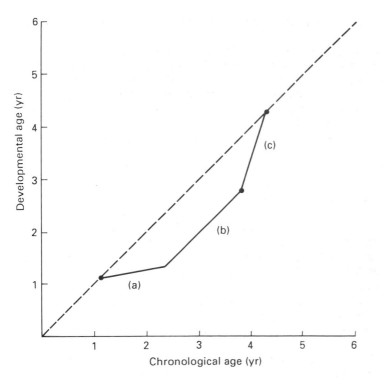

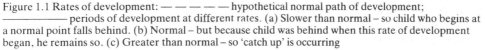

Figure 1.1 Rates of development: — — — — — hypothetical normal path of development; ——————— periods of development at different rates. (a) Slower than normal – so child who begins at a normal point falls behind. (b) Normal – but because child was behind when this rate of development began, he remains so. (c) Greater than normal – so 'catch up' is occurring

disabled child is handicapped is determined by the demands of his environment. Likewise, the exposure of a normal healthy child to unfavourable circumstances of sufficient severity for long enough may produce permanent disability which will persist even when the environmental stresses are corrected.

A *deprived* child is one who, for any reason, is deprived of a normal home life and who in consequence needs the temporary or permanent care or protection of a recognized child care agency. According to Sheridan this definition, in contrast to the others, is official and of legal significance.

Disorder, defect, deformity, impairment, disability, handicap

Each of these terms has a precise meaning (WHO, 1980); all too often they are used loosely and interchangeably to the disadvantage of children and parents, and confusion of the professionals:

1. *Disorder*: an illness or structural defect. The context will show which meaning applies. If the latter, then the term is synonymous with defect.
2. *Defect*: abnormality of structure.

3. *Deformity*: deviation from the normal shape and form.
4. *Impairment*: loss or abnormality of psychological, physiological or anatomical structure or function usually synonymous with disability, but may also be used in place of defect or damage.
5. *Disability*: failure of function or skill.
6. *Handicap*: impediment to an individual's development, opportunities, expectations and activities.

The adjectival form of defect, defective, is often used loosely to describe impairment of function and not just abnormality of structure. Thus, 'a defective ear drum', meaning one which is abnormal and perforated, is an appropriate use of the word, whereas 'defective hearing', meaning impairment of hearing without necessarily any structural abnormality, may be misleading, and 'hearing disability' or 'impairment' are preferable terms.

Deformity is used particularly in connection with acquired abnormalities which arise during the course of an illness, e.g. equinus deformity in cerebral palsy.

Defects and deformities may give rise to disability, but need not necessarily do so. Many who see children with defects and deformities assume that they will be disabled and so may underestimate their capabilities. Whereas children who are disabled and also have obvious defects excite sympathy, those who are disabled but otherwise appear healthy and fit may suffer because no one understands their difficulties. Children with 'hidden' disabilities such as a communication disorder can suffer greatly in this way.

During the course of a long-term disorder such as cerebral palsy, the degrees of deformity and disability may change in opposite directions, with one improving while the other becomes worse. For example, a child with cerebral palsy may increase his speed and distance of walking and so considerably reduce his disability, but the muscular effort required to achieve this improvement may result in an increase in deformity. This situation produces considerable therapeutic dilemmas (Holt, 1963).

A disabled child may be handicapped, but there is neither a direct nor a close relationship between the extent of disability and associated handicap. The extent to which a child is handicapped depends not only upon the nature and extent of the disability, but also upon the significance of the disability to the child and the success or otherwise with which the child can by-pass or compensate for the disability. For example, the extent to which a child with disability of the hands is handicapped depends, among other things, upon his drive to overcome his limitations and the amount he is required to do with his hands. Literature contains many examples of individuals with considerable disabilities who were able, nevertheless, to lead very full, productive and satisfying lives. Far from handicapping them, their difficulties seemed to spur them to ever greater achievements. It should not be assumed that a disabled child will be handicapped. One should never adopt a negative and pessimistic outlook towards such children.

The qualifying word *multiple* is often associated with the terms defect, deformity, disability and handicap. A child may have several of these problems, so it is quite appropriate for the word multiple to be added. But the addition of 'multiple' to one of these terms should not be transferred automatically to the other terms. For example, a child with multiple defects may suffer only a single disability. Thus a child with defects in various parts of the body, such as malformed ears, congenital heart defect and lower limb deficiency, may be disabled only with respect to walking, whereas a child with a single disability such as severe hearing impairment may be multiply handicapped, e.g. educationally, emotionally and socially.

References

Black, D. (1980) *Inequalities in Health*. London: DHSS/HMSO

Holt, K. S. (1963) Deformity and disability in cerebral palsy. *Devl. Med. Child Neurol.*, **5,** 629

Sheridan, M. D. (1962) Infants at risk of handicapping conditions. *Mon. Bull. Minist. Hlth* **21**, 238

Sheridan, M. D. (1969) Definitions relating to developmental paediatrics. *Hlth Trends*, DHSS, **1**, 2,5

WHO (1980) *International Classification of Impairments, Disabilities and Handicaps*. Geneva: World Health Organisation

Chapter 2

Neural maturation

Growth of the brain

It is axiomatic that many of the features of human development are dependent upon and occur as a result of development of the brain. The brief synopsis of brain development which follows cannot possibly do justice to all that takes place as the brain grows, differentiates and matures, but it will perhaps convey an impression of the magnitude and complexity of the processes involved.

The easily observed increase of head size with age demonstrates growth of the brain. On those occasions when the brain itself can be inspected, the increasing complexity of its structure with advancing age is readily apparent. These, however, are crude manifestations of the brain's growth, and all the vital changes occur at cellular level. Knowledge of brain development at cellular level is increasing as a result of careful studies of the histological, chemical and electrical features of the brain, and considerable advances can be anticipated in the coming years.

Gross structural development

The growth of the brain is reflected in the increase of head size with age. The clinician's most useful guide to this growth is measurement of the head circumference. The measurement is made with an accurately marked, non-stretchable, narrow tape passed firmly around the head just above the bridge of the nose and over the occipital prominence, as shown in Figure 2.1.

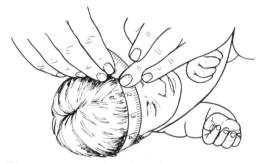

Figure 2.1 Measurement of head circumference of a baby

The measurements are used in two ways:

1. They are compared with standard data to determine whether the head circumference deviates markedly from that expected for the age of the child. It is useful to know the source of the data so as to be satisfied that it was collected from a suitable population and is reliable. The data should be expressed either in centiles or as mean and standard deviations.
2. Serial measurements are plotted on a graph to show the changes with age.

Two graphs are usually needed, one covering the period from mid-fetal life to about 2 years of age, and the other covering the period from about 3 years to adulthood.

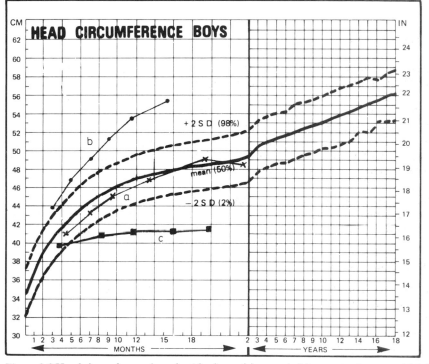

Figure 2.2 Head circumference/age chart for boys: (a) normal; (b) excessive increase; (c) failure of increase

Figure 2.2 shows a head circumference/age chart which has been found to be satisfactory for general use (Nellhaus, 1968). Three sets of measurements are shown to illustrate the following:

(a) Initial and subsequent measurements all within the expected range – a normal child with normal brain growth.
(b) Initial measurements greater than expectation and subsequent measurements showing an excessively high rate of growth – a child suffering from hydrocephalus.
(c) Initial measurement within the expected range, but subsequent measurements fall below expectation – slowing of brain growth in a moderately retarded child.

Some variation of head circumference occurs between different ethnic groups, but this is not very large, and certainly is not great enough to justify the almost impossible task of producing separate charts for each ethnic group.

More significant variations of head circumference occur with body weight, so allowances should be made if the infant is much bigger or smaller than expected for his age (Illingworth and Lutz, 1965). The following is a useful working rule:

1. *Babies under 6 months of age.* Allow 1.3 cm in the head circumference for each kg deviation of body weight from the mean.
2. *Babies aged 6–12 months.* Allow 1.0 cm in the head circumference for each kg deviation of body weight from the mean.

At birth the human brain is about half its adult size. It increases rapidly to about three-quarters of adult size by 18 months of age, and 90% by 4 years of age. By this later age the rate of growth has slowed considerably and the remaining 10% of growth occurs gradually throughout childhood.

Gross structural differentiation

In the early stages of growth of the brain it is possible to identify five major parts. These are the fore-, mid- and hind-brains, and the cerebral hemispheres and cerebellum. The fore-, mid- and hind-brains appear as distinct bulbar swellings of the initial tubular cell mass which constitutes the primitive brain. These then become overlaid by the mantle of the cerebral hemispheres, and the cerebellum appears as a mid-line posterior structure (Figure 2.3). This structural differentiation of the brain occurs during the first trimester of pregnancy. As early as 10 weeks the five major parts of the primitive brain can be identified despite the fact that the embryo is still quite small – little more than 15 mm in length and weighing only 20–30 g. Any disturbance of the growth of the brain in this early stage is likely to produce serious malformations such as anencephaly and spina bifida.

During the second trimester of pregnancy the brain increases rapidly in size. Most noticeable upon inspection is the increase of the cerebral hemispheres which appear to be appreciably larger each week. Throughout most of this period, however, the hemispheres remain smooth. In contrast, the third trimester is characterized by the appearance of indentations and convolutions of the cerebral cortex. Figure 2.4 shows the typical appearance of the developing brain at successive stages of fetal life.

Cellular development

The important features of cellular development are proliferation, migration, differentiation, dendritic formation and synaptic connection.

Cellular development follows an orderly sequence. First, neuroblasts proliferate in several germinative zones in the sub-ependymal, sub-pia-arachnoid and periventricular areas. This process begins early in pregnancy and is complete before birth, by which time the brain has total complement of neurones.

Proliferation of the cells is followed by migration and functional differentiation. Cellular migration is one of the most remarkable features of brain development. It appears to be a self-organizing process which is guided by the characteristics of the cell membranes (Herschkowitz and Rossi, 1972). The characteristics of the cell membranes and the appearance and disappearance of several enzymes at

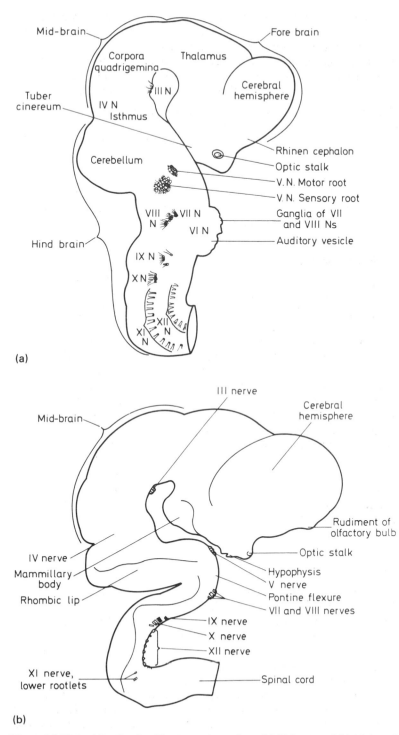

(a)

(b)

Figure 2.3 Right side of brain of human embryo about (a) 10.2 mm and (b) 13.6 mm long

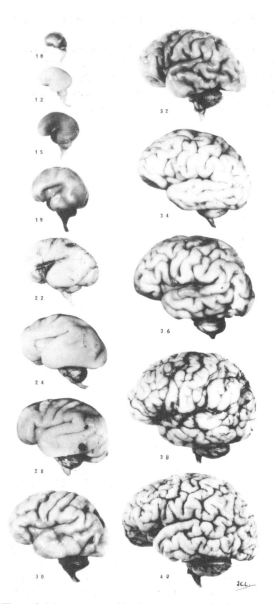

Figure 2.4 Appearance of brain at successive fetal ages (age in weeks shown by figures)

appropriate stages are regulated by genetic influences (Paigen, 1971; Baurlacher, 1973). Cellular migration and differentiation begins in the 3rd month of pregnancy and continues to term. The cells migrate from their origin in successive concentric layers, long thin chains, or clusters until they reach their destination where they assume the distinctive features and functions for cells in that particular area. In this way distinctive cell agglomerations appear as nuclei and bands. The rapidity with which these changes occur may be judged from the fact that in human fetuses the cerebral cortex is just identifiable at 10 weeks, yet by 26 weeks it is well developed with all six cellular layers evident.

The extent of migration is illustrated by the anatomy of the seventh nerve. The nucleus of the facial nerve forms under the floor of the fourth ventricle slightly proximal and dorsal to the nucleus of the sixth (abducens) nerve. Then, in relation to the sixth nucleus it migrates dorsally, medially and caudally, and then sweeps ventrolaterally. As a result the tract of the facial nerve follows a long arc-like course around the sixth nerve nucleus before emerging from the ventral surface of the pons (Figure 2.5).

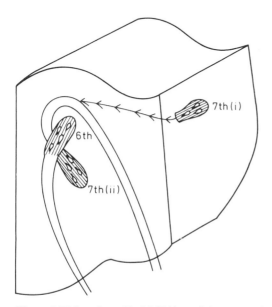

Figure 2.5 Migration of facial (7th) cranial nerve nucleus. Diagram shows a portion of the pons indicating the initial position of the 7th nerve nucleus (i), and the final tracts of the 6th and 7th nerves (ii)

The proliferation, migration and differentiation of neurones in the developing human brain occur during the second and third trimesters. Although some glial cells are formed during fetal life, it is in the months immediately following birth when these cells proliferate. Dendritic elaboration occurs very actively at the same time. Myelination begins early (about 22 weeks) in the spinal cord roots, and by birth there is some evidence of myelination in almost all parts of the central nervous system. The peak period of myelination, however, occurs postnatally, after the peak activity of glial formation.

Although the sequences of cellular development are related to birth as a convenient time marker, they are not dependent on birth.

The function of the central nervous system depends upon the synaptic connections between the axons and dendrites of cells. In order to achieve the correct connections it is thought that cellular development is excessive and that alongside the progressive changes there is regression of superfluous material with death of neurones and retraction of axons (Greenough, Black and Wallace, 1987).

There is interesting speculation about the control of these processes. What determines which connections survive and which disappear? Is it all predetermined, or does experience with use of the connections play a part?

As a consequence of these studies and speculations Greenough, Black and Wallace (1987) propose a new scheme for the relationship between experience and brain function. Two processes are described. *Experience-expectant information storage* refers to experiences common to all members of the species. Neural development occurs in expectation of these experiences and when they occur the pattern of neural connections is established. *Experience-dependent information storage* refers to experiences unique to each individual. Neural development then occurs as an active process in response to these experiences.

This hypothesis offers an opportunity to review the concepts of critical and sensitive periods (see later) and the potential for stimulating experience-dependent changes in development and behaviour.

The rapidly developing brain requires an abundant supply of energy and nutrients. Although knowledge about the metabolism of the growing brain is still being obtained, it is clear that many biological features and adjustments enable it to obtain the energy it requires during this vulnerable period. For example, there may be qualitative as well as quantitative differences between the proteins and enzymes of the growing brain as compared with the mature brain (Sterman, McGinty and Adinolfi, 1971); the blood-brain barrier matures at different times for different substances (Myers and Bito, 1973); and ketones may play an exceptionally important role in the metabolism of the growing brain (Wilkinson and Buckley, 1973).

The developing brain is susceptible to the effects of nutritional deprivation. Dobbing and Sands (1973), Dobbing (1974) and Dobbing and Stuart (1974) hypothesize that such deprivation would be expected to have the greatest impact upon the most rapidly growing tissues at that particular time. For example, intra-uterine nutritional deprivation might be expected to have the greatest effect upon the neurones, whereas postnatal deprivation would affect glial cells, myelination, and dendritic processes.

There is much still to be learnt about brain growth and development and many can make some contribution. The developmental paediatrician may feel that his clinical observations cannot match the sophisticated investigative methods of the cellular physiologist and biochemist. He must realize, however, that there are limits both to the understanding of human brain development from studies upon other species and the opportunities for investigations upon humans. In these circumstances careful developmental observations and clinical analysis may provide clues to improve our understanding of brain function. For the present, it is as well to remember how far we have still to go and to be aware of our present limitations.

Electrical changes

One of the few ways of exploring the activity of the functioning human brain is by recording and analysing the electrical potentials which come from it. Considerable skill and much experience is needed. The problems which have to be overcome include devising ways of making intra-uterine recordings from the fetus; increasing the effectiveness of transabdominal recordings; and trying to ensure that anything recorded represents true brain activity and is not due to brain damage or anoxia. Dreyfuss-Brisac (1966) described the appearance of electrical activity in the brain.

She considers that the electroencephalogram correlates closely with the stage of maturation of the brain. The characteristic patterns are as follows:

Conceptual age (weeks)	Characteristic pattern
24–28	Discontinuous tracing with polymorphic rhythms, but without organized features. Bursts of very slow waves (0.3–1.0 Hz and 5–6 Hz. Occasional spikes.
28–32	A simpler pattern than earlier with long quiet periods and 1–2 s bursts of regular theta activity of 4–6 Hz and amplitudes of 25–100 µV.
32–37	The record now shows more continuous activity, especially in the occipital areas. Delta waves of 10–14 Hz are present.
37–41	Differences between the sleeping and awake records are present for the first time. The awake records show a continuous pattern. In light sleep the pattern resembles that of the earlier stage, whereas with deep sleep the pattern becomes discontinuous, paroxysmal and asynergic.

A visually evoked response can be obtained from 50% of newborns. It shows a longer latency and higher potential than a typical adult record. When the response is obtained from prematures, the initial phase is usually absent and the latency is even longer. It is said that the length of the latent period correlates with the conceptual age (Hobek, Karlsberg and Olsson, 1973).

In the auditory field most interest has been in the evoked responses from the brainstem. Several distinct waveforms can be identified and the latency time of their appearance decreases with maturation of the brain. The changes are most marked during the 24th to 34th week of gestation (Roberts, Davis and Phon, 1982).

References

Baurlacher, K. E. (1973) Developmental aspects of amino acid transport. In *Inborn Errors of Metabolism* (eds. Hommes, F. A. and van der Berg, C. J.). London: Academic Press

Dobbing, J. (1974) The later development of the brain and its vulnerability. In *Scientific Foundations of Paediatrics* (eds. Davis, J. A. and Dobbing, J.). London: Heinemann

Dobbing, J. and Sands, J. (1973) Quantitative growth and development of the human brain. *Archs Dis. Childh.*, **48**, 747

Dobbing, J. and Stuart, J. L. (1974) Vulnerability of developing brain and behaviour. *Br. Med. Bull.*, **30**, 1164

Dreyfuss-Brisac, C. (1966) The bioelectrical development of the central nervous system during early life. In *Human Development* (ed. Falkner, F.). Philadelphia: Saunders

Greenough, W. T., Black, J. E. and Wallace, C. S. (1987) Experience and brain development. *Child Development*, **58**, 539–559

Herschkowitz, N. and Rossi, E. (1972) Critical periods of brain development. In *Lipids, Malnutrition and the Developing Brain*. Ciba Foundation Symposium. London: Associated Science Publications.

Hobek, A., Karlsberg, P. and Olsson, J. (1973) Development of visual and somatosensory evoked responses in pre-term newborn infants. *Electroenceph. Clin. Neurophysiol.*, **34**, 225

Illingworth, R. S. and Lutz, W. (1965) Head circumference of infants related to body weight. *Archs Dis. Childh.*, **40**, 672

Myers, R. E. and Bito, L. Z. (1973) Ontogenesis of blood-brain barrier function in primate: CSF cation regulations. In *Fetal and Neonatal Physiology*, Barcroft Centenary Symposium. Cambridge: Cambridge University Press

Nellhaus, G. (1968) Composite international and inter-racial graphs. *Pediatrics*, **41**, 106

Paigen, K. (1971) Enzyme systems and degradation. In *Mammalian Systems* (ed. Recheigl, M.). Washington D. C.: Karger

Roberts, J. L., Davis, H. and Phon, G. L. (1982) Auditory brainstem reponses in pre-term neonates. Maturation and follow-up. *J. Pediatr.,* **10**, 257

Sterman, M. B., McGinty, D. J. and Adinolfi, A. M. (1971) *Brain Development and Behaviour.* London: Academic Press

Wilkinson, D. H. and Buckley, B. M. (1973) Role of ketone bodies in brain development. In *Inborn Errors of Metabolism* (eds. Hommes, F. A. and van der Berg, C. J.). London: Academic Press

Chapter 3

Some theories of child development

Many approach the subject of child development with a belief that it is simple and uncomplicated, but this is far from the truth. The 'obviousness' of child development and belief in its simplicity probably go a long way towards accounting for the relative sparseness of original research in the subject. There are notable exceptions, but on the whole child development has not received the attention of research workers which it requires and deserves. Several hypotheses about development have been put forward, but until recent years little sound experimental work had been carried out to substantiate or refute them.

Although it is not yet possible to put forward a complete theory of development and a clear explanation of all the mechanisms involved, it is profitable, nevertheless, to examine some of the views which have been propounded. Doing so should provide a deeper understanding of child development, and may also cause us to review our own current views about development. Such an exercise is especially valuable because, whatever views one has, however incomplete, they will profoundly influence our attitudes towards children.

No attempt is made to provide a comprehensive review of all the theories of child development. Mention will be made of four important and very influential views, and an attempt will be made to summarize the present situation. It is hoped that this attempt will provide clinicians with a perspective and a basis for understanding child development, and will stimulate them to explore the subject further.

All theories of child development lie between two extremes. On the one hand there is the idea that the infant is completely naive and his brain is like an empty sheet. Every character and thought has to be introduced by indoctrination and training, and learning and experiences are engraved upon the blank sheet of the brain. In the past, such views led to some very harsh training routines for young children, but at the present time such extreme opinions are not widely held.

On the other hand there is the view that all abilities and understanding are contained within the brain, and that as the brain grows there is a gradual unfolding of a predetermined pattern of development. This view emphasizes the inherent capacity of the nervous system and denies the influence of environmental experience. Maturation is all! This view was supported by the work of Gesell; it received much support in the earlier part of this century and still has some adherents. Adoption of this outlook leads to a passive attitude towards children with developmental difficulties. It is assumed that they will be capable of performing the missing abilities when the brain is sufficiently mature, and that in the meantime nothing need be done.

Neither of these two extreme views is acceptable today. Arguments about the relative importance of nature and nurture which these considerations provoke are not very fruitful. What is required is an appreciation of all the mechanisms concerned in human development. As our understanding of these increases we begin to realize that the maturation of the nervous system and the results of external experience are intertwined and interrelated. It is hoped that a consideration of some of the major theories of child development will lead the way to an acceptable synthesis of the various views.

Gesell's approach to child development (e.g. Gesell et al., 1930; Gesell and Amatruda, 1947; Gesell, 1948, 1966)

Arnold Gesell was the founder of the Child Development Center at Yale University and its inspiration for many years. He and his colleagues observed and recorded the responses and behaviour of babies and children when they were placed in standard prearranged situations. Their subsequent detailed analysis of the cine film and written records form the basis of their descriptions, statements of principles, and hypotheses about the mechanisms of child development.

Their descriptions of child development are as vivid and comprehensive as any which exist. They recognized that various responses and behaviour patterns emerged gradually. Some responses are of a *permanent* nature; that is, once they have appeared they persist as a constant feature of the child's behavioural repertoire. Failure of such items to appear at the expected ages indicates delayed development.

Other responses are of a *temporary* nature in that they appear for a period and then are superseded by another type of response. Failure to observe a temporary type of response at the appropriate age may indicate: (a) delay in development – the response appears later; (b) accelerated development, in which case the temporary item was present earlier and has been superseded already; (c) weakness of the response so that it is overlooked.

Gesell described the features of development as it occurred in several channels or pathways, thus: gross and fine motor, adaptive, language and personal–social pathways. This separation assists in the analysis of observed development and has been followed, with various modifications, by many subsequent workers. He emphasized that, despite the usefulness of such a separation into pathways, in order to obtain an understanding of child development it was necessary to appreciate its integrated wholeness and its flowing continuity.

On the basis of his observations Gesell considered the pattern of development to be so uniform that he felt that it must follow several principles: (a) development follows a definite sequence; (b) development shows a cephalocaudal progression; (c) development proceeds from gross undifferentiated skills to precise and refined ones.

These aspects were considered to be relatively immutable. Many subsequent workers interpreted these principles as laws which every child must obey, and this led to recommendations that children who show variations in their development must be made to repeat earlier developmental sequences in the 'correct' order so as to develop normally.

The one aspect of development which Gesell accepted might vary was its rate, which was slowed in certain conditions and circumstances.

Gesell was a paediatrician who wrote for paediatricians in order to help them in their clinical work. Consequently, having described the observed stages of development and defined the principles of development, it was a relatively short step to the concept of developmental diagnosis. The major abnormality which may be diagnosed is, of course *developmental delay*, but other types of developmental abnormality to be found are: (a) *an abnormal quality of performance;* (b) *the undue persistence of temporary responses;* (c) *a disordered sequence of development.*

Another type of abnormality, *developmental dissociation*, has been described by Illingworth, an ardent follower of Gesell (Illingworth, 1958).

Gesell considered that the observed developmental phenomena reflected maturation of the central nervous system. This hypothesis received much support from observations and experiments which were being reported about this time. These experiments fall into two categories. One group is concerned with evidence that responses and actions develop despite restraint. Observations were made on children who were swaddled (Greenacre, 1944), anaesthetized tadpoles (Carmichael, 1926) and restrained birds (Dennis, 1943). In all these cases the children walked, the tadpoles swam, and the birds flew when released. The interpretation made from these observations was that maturation of the nervous system had continued during the period of restraint so that the particular skill was there and ready for use at the appropriate time. Development thus depended upon maturation. These studies did not examine in any depth the quality of performance of the skills in these circumstances, the effect of the restraint upon other aspects of development, or the developmental value of the experiences which the individual would have undergone had he not been restrained. The studies show that maturation of the nervous system is important in the development of motor skills, but it is unjustified, on the basis of this evidence, to conclude that maturation is the only influence of importance in the development of motor skills, or of all other aspects of development.

The other group of observations is concerned with evidence that practice prior to the usual time of appearance of a particular skill does not hasten its appearance. Several studies were reported in which one member of a set of identical twins was given early training and practice, and when both twins were examined at a later age the untrained one possessed the same motor skills as the trained one (Gesell and Thompson, 1929; McGraw, 1935). The interpretation of these observations was that abilities develop irrespective of training and when the nervous system is ready for them to do so. Therefore, development is dependent upon maturation of the nervous system. These are undoubtedly important observations and it is reasonable to accept that a certain level of neurological function is necessary for a particular ability to be possible, but the conclusions have been applied more widely and rigidly than is justified. They have been responsible for a very widespread negative attitude among clinicians towards therapy for young handicapped children. It is maintained that nothing need to be done to help a child showing delayed or aberrant development because the missing abilities will appear as the brain matures. This attitude assumes that:

(a) the results of relatively crude observations upon a few healthy twins apply to all children and in all circumstances;
(b) when the nervous system has reached a level of maturity appropriate for the appearance of a particular ability, this ability will manifest itself whatever the circumstances;

(c) no attention is necessary to ensure the persistence and elaboration of any ability once it appears.

For these reasons I find it difficult to accept the strong views arising from Gesell's work about the futility of treatment of young disabled children.

The weaknesses of the Gesell approach to development are that it does not include sufficient experimental work to back up the conclusions drawn from the excellent descriptions, that it emphasizes the motor aspects of development more than the others, and that it is too rigidly adherent to the concept of maturation.

The strengths of the Gesell approach to development lie in its wealth of accurate clinical descriptions, the concept of the dynamic continuity of development, and its clinical applicability to developmental diagnosis.

The Gesell approach to child development appeals particularly to clinicians; Piaget's approach (see below) appeals particularly to educationalists.

Piaget's contribution to child development (Flavell, 1963; Brearley and Hitchfield, 1967; Maier, 1969)

Piaget, a Swiss, trained initially as a zoologist, but later turned to psychology. He revolutionized thinking about cognitive development in childhood. His work is based upon extremely detailed and precise observations of children, especially his own children, the results of which he then subjected to intense logical reasoning and, following this, he tested his conclusions in simple experimental ways.

He was interested in the cause and effect of every action and every response. He wanted to find out what the responses meant to the child and how they helped him to adapt to his environment, because he considered such adaptation to be a fundamental feature of development. His methods and reasoning will be understood better by considering the steps taken in the acquisition of a mature concept of an object.

A mature object concept consists of 'seeing' it as an entity in its own right, existing and moving in space and persisting in time. The object exists independently of any activity on the part of the observer, or other person, such as looking at it, manipulating it, smelling it or listening to it. As an individual conceptualizes objects as separate entities in this mature way, he also conceives object-like properties in respect to himself. Piaget described the following stages through which children reached this mature concept:

Stages 1 and 2. The object presents sensory impressions which may be 'sensed' by the child. Continued looking (or touching, smelling or listening to) is encouraged by the pleasure evoked by the sensory impressions, which may persist after the object is moved.

Stage 3. The child begins to extrapolate in time and space by a series of manoeuvres: (a) he shows visual anticipation of movements of the object; (b) he searches for the object. Visually this is a roving search over the whole immediate area; (c) he plays with a 'there – not there' situation – he looks at the object, then turns away, then looks back at the object again, and does this repeatedly; (d) he anticipates the whole object when seeing only a part; (e) he will remove an obstruction to see the object.

Stage 4. He searches for hidden objects with increasing degrees of sophistication.
Stage 5. He focuses his search upon the place where the object was last seen.
Stage 6. He searches for objects by imagining a series of possible positions which
they might be occupying. In this way he demonstrates his awareness that objects
have an existence apart from himself.

These conclusions are drawn from numerous careful observations like this one:

> At 0.7 (months) Jacqueline tries to grasp a celluloid duck on top of her quilt. She almost
> catches it, shakes herself, and the duck slides down beside her. It falls very close to her
> hand but behind a fold in the sheet. Jacqueline's eyes have followed the movement, she
> has even followed it with her outstretched hand. But as soon as the duck has disappeared –
> nothing more. It does not occur to her to search behind the fold of the sheet, which would
> be very easy to do (she twists it mechanically without searching at all).

The simple but very neat experimental studies devised by Piaget and his
colleagues can be illustrated by describing the investigation of understanding of
quantity. The examiner makes a ball of clay and the subject makes another one just
like it. One ball is kept as a standard of reference and the other is distorted in
various ways. The child is then asked if it is the same substance, same weight and
same volume. Experiments of this type revealed that at first there is no sense of
conservation of matter, volume or weight; then occurs a transitional period during
which some transformations are recognized; and then finally comes a stage when all
transformations are recognized. Appreciation of conservation of matter becomes
common at 8–10 years, of weight at 10–12 years and of volume only after 12 years.

Piaget and co-workers accumulated a vast amount of data upon which they based
descriptions of the processes and patterns of development of cognitive reasoning in
infancy and childhood. Development is considered to occur as a result of the
interaction of four processes:

1. *Maturation.* Differentiation and elaboration of the central nervous system.
2. *Experience.* Interaction with the physical world.
3. *Social transmission.* The effect of care and education upon the nature of
   experience.
4. *Equilibration.* Self-regulation.

The essence of development is seen in a biological sense as the individual's
adaptation to his environment. In development, differentiation is made between
two aspects of adaptation, namely (a) *assimilation* which consists of an individual's
ability to accept and integrate experiences; (b) *accommodation* which consists of
the modifications provoked by experiences.

For example, a cube placed in front of a baby provides visual and tactile stimuli
which are assimilated, and they provoke visual regard, manipulation and mouthing
as accommodative responses.

Development is a continuous process built up stage by stage in a developmental
hierarchy. Time is required for each process to be practised, to be perfected, and
then used as the basis for the next succeeding stage.

This method of thinking about development led to the differentiation of
horizontal and *vertical* features. When a new task appears which requires the same
level of organization as an earlier one, a horizontal expansion of development is
said to have taken place; but when a new task appears which requires a higher level
of organization than previously, this is said to be vertical development.

Development is dynamic in that a child is never anything, but is always becoming something. Actions are important in Piagetian development since they are the expression of cerebral processes, whereas thoughts are essentially internalized actions.

Piaget and his co-workers showed that each reasoning process leads on to the next more complex one. They described the following stages, each of which contains several substages, and arranged them in chronological sequence.

Sensorimotor stage (up to approximately 2 years)

In a sense this period of development involves the whole infant. He is coming to grips with his physical world – learning to deal with sensory experiences, fulfilling his physical needs, and using his whole self for expression and communication. During this period the infant learns to perceive his environment and to control his actions. The substages are as follows:

(a) Use of reflex actions (0–1 month).
(b) Development of habituation of actions (1–4 months).

A response is repeated until it becomes an established schema. This is the beginning of repetition in sequence. The repetition of a response is called a *circular action*. The actions which develop during this period are called *primary circular reactions*. These lead to the appearance of the first voluntary action.

(c) Co-ordination of actions (4–8 months), e.g. vision and pre-hension.

The primary circular reactions are now extended beyond the immediate basic needs to have a secondary function, now called *secondary circular reactions*, which opens up the possibility of developing imitation, play and emotion.

(d) Co-ordination of secondary schemata in which previous experiences are used to influence actions (8–12 months).

This is an important transitional substage. The child's greater mobility is an important influence. This stage opens up new dimensions such as ability to recognize signs, to anticipate response, and to observe.

(e) Differentiation of action schemata in which new ways are found by experimentation (12–18 months).

The circular reactions are further developed to a *tertiary stage* in which repetitions are modified when new objects are met and are further modified to explore the object purposefully.

(f) Internalization of schemata in which all the earliest reactions become incorporated into automatic spontaneous responses (18 months onwards).

The last substage (f) is the third and most complex of the goal-directed behaviour responses seen in the period of sensorimotor development. The first was seen in substage (d) and consisted of the co-ordination of existing and familiar schemata. The second was seen in substage (e) and consisted of experimentation to discover new ways to use existing schemata. In substage (e) possible solutions to new situations are worked out internally before being put to the test. Existing schemata are now internalized and the most appropriate one is selected to deal with new challenges. At this time the child also becomes aware of the independent existence of objects and to some extent of his own identity. These are vital changes for the development of his personality and social relationships.

Stage of concrete operations (from approximately 2 to 12 years)

The study of concrete operations in cognitive development from 6 to 12 years is one of the most complete aspects of Piaget's work. The preceding years of preparation and transition also possess much richness of their own, with the development of symbolization, language, play and personality being important parts.

(a) Symbolic function: pre-conceptual (2–4 years).

At this substage the child knows the world as he sees it and experiences it. He lives in the here and now and knows no alternatives. The sensorimotor stage equipped him to explore further as he does in constant play. He is further helped in this by recognizing that objects may be represented by models or can be identified in various ways, most particularly by verbal symbols.

(b) Intuitive thought (4–7 years):
    (i) representational organization;
    (ii) articulated representational regulations.

The child's world expands considerably at this age. He starts school; he has many playmates. He relies upon imitation of the behaviour of others (especially adults) to deal with many new experiences. It is as if he intuitively knew what to do, but all the time he is learning. He replaces acting-out of his thoughts and reasoning with talking-out; much of his play is verbally controlled. Much of this period is occupied with learning how to deal with an increasing number of concepts and to order them in place and time. Language is an essential help in this process. It is used as a tool of intuitive thought, to help to order the various concepts and to deal with social relationships.

(c) Concrete operations (6–12 years):
    (i) simple operations, e.g. classification;
    (ii) whole systems operations, e.g. co-ordinates.

This is the period during which the child achieves mastery over his physical world. He has learnt about many properties possessed by objects in his environment and now he begins to compare and contrast different objects and to classify them. He recognizes the relationships of parts to the whole, and he groups similar items together in time and space. To deal with all this information the child develops a series of logical strategies of increasing complexity.

Stage of formal operations (approximately 12 years onwards)

(a) Hypothesis-deductive operations.
(b) Lattice operations.

The characteristics of this stage of Piagetian development are the replacement of random cognitive behaviour by a systematic approach to problems, and the acquisition of abilities to hypothesize, to reason deductively and to understand and work out complex interrelationships. Understanding of the physical properties of objects has proceeded in the sequence (i) space, time, reality and causation; (ii) number, order, measure, shape and size; (iii) motion, speed, force and energy.

The experiences of past opportunities to compare and contrast have led to concepts of equality and balance between concepts and actions. This understanding is applied to social relationships as well as to physical entities and underlies much of the awakening of personal awareness which characterizes adolescence.

It is quite impossible to do justice to all of Piaget's thinking in this brief summary, but I hope sufficient has been written to show that this is more than just a description of observed development. It is an exploration in depth of the processes involved in the child's cognitive reasoning. Its great value is that it provides an insight into the child's strategies of problem-solving and provides a sound basis for developmental intervention and teaching programmes. It does not cover all aspects of development, and it has been criticized for not taking more account of the Freudian views of childhood. That Piaget did consider this aspect is reflected in his writings. It is possible that the detailed analysis of cognitive reasoning does not readily lend itself to psychoanalytical appreciation, which requires an understanding of the global effects of experience. For this we need to turn to the appropriate literature.

Psychoanalytical approach to child development with particular reference to Erikson's concepts (Winnicott, 1957; Erikson, 1967; Maier, 1969)

Freud and his followers revealed those strong influences, of which we are not normally aware, which control our emotional development and stability, attitudes and reactions, and interpersonal relationships. They showed the continuity of these influences, and demonstrated that early childhood experiences may have profound consequences later on. Their studies showed that the direction of the child's psychic orientation changes at different ages. Thus, in the first year there is a predominance of an oral orientation; of elimination (or anal–urethral) orientation in the second and third years; and of sexual (or genital) orientation in later years.

The vast literature on these subjects cannot possibly be covered in this brief review. Nevertheless, there is much in the psychoanalytical literature which is pertinent to child development and of which developmental paediatricians should be aware. Some familiarity with the writings of Anna Freud and of Donald Winnicott would serve as a sound beginning. The latter's popular lectures of the early 1940s on child-rearing are excellent reading for practising paediatricians.

The work of Erikson has been selected for further comment because he of all psychoanalysts has ordered his views towards an understanding of child development.

Following a sound training in Freudian concepts Erikson moved from Europe to America where he added to his psychoanalytical views additional information derived from observations of children, anthropological data, and studies of child-rearing practices. He then elaborated his ideas into a theory of child development. Erikson believes the following to be important for children:

(a) to have an awareness and stability which is appropriate for their level of development;

(b) that this awareness and stability is achieved by balancing opposing influences, and that behaviour at any age is a reflection of their success in achieving this balance;
(c) that the direction of the orientation of their equilibrium varies at different ages;
(e) that periods of transition from one orientation to another are times of crisis and stress.

Erikson describes the following five phases during childhood.

Infancy – sense of trust

The infant is vulnerable and needs to acquire a sense of security and trust. The unfamiliarity of everything around him creates uncertainty and mistrust. He is very dependent upon all the strengths derived from the mothering situation to balance the contrary doubts and so achieve equilibrium. His attractiveness and dependency help him to acquire stability by provoking strong feelings of tenderness in those who care for him.

Early childhood – sense of autonomy

Awareness of his own will stimulates a child to exercise it to create a sense of autonomy. This positive drive forwards is associated with apprehension about the strength of his will and shame over abandoning the ties of phase 1, thereby setting the scene for the conflicts of phase 2. The environment created by his parents is important; if too restrictive the child cannot exercise his own will; if too permissive the child overstretches himself and creates anxiety. The child strives to achieve a balance within his particular personal environment.

Pre-school – sense of initiative

Having a sense of autonomy, and coming to believe that he is what he thinks he is, he now explores new worlds in which he tests himself. He begins to join in other children's activities, as is well seen by observing young children at play. His drive to initiate activities, to explore and to exert himself meets rebuffs and causes frustration. This conflicting situation often extends into his rich fantasy world where many problems are worked out. The efforts of the struggle to achieve a balance may provoke resentment and rebellion against trusted parents who let him get into this situation.

School age – sense of industry

By school age the child has reached a stage of considerable physical and intellectual energies which he applies in order to master all he can. A school child is receptive to all he is taught and responds accordingly. Contrary influences consist of a fear of failure and a sense of inferiority with respect to his peers. He struggles to achieve a balance between industry and inferiority in his intellectual and physical pursuits and his social relationships.

Adolescence – sense of identity

The individual now moves forward to reach a readiness to face the entire world. On the one hand there is his awareness of his many abilities and skills and confidence in them, and on the other hand there is his awareness of the many uncertainties in the world and a reluctance to plunge ahead on his own. Some of the conflicts of this period, as identified by Erikson, are as follows:

(a) time perspective and acceptance in contrast to time diffusion – doing the good things on time, hoping the bad things will never come;
(b) self-certainty in contrast to self-uncertainty and self-consciousness;
(c) acceptance or evasion of roles and identities;
(d) persistence in anticipation of achievement in contrast to sporadic activity with periods of work paralysis;
(e) sexual identification and acceptance in contrast to bisexual diffusion and conflicts;
(f) leadership versus diffusion of authority.
(g) uncompromising idealogical polarization in contrast to tolerance for diffusion of ideals.

Erikson's approach to child development creates an impression of a dynamic situation, and it provides clinicians, especially child psychiatrists and paediatricians, with a structure which can be the basis of therapeutic intervention. For example, his views of basic trust in phase 1, a trust which needs to be achieved by all babies, help one to understand the difficulties of a malformed baby who cannot find that security from his distraught mother. This then provides a basis for therapeutic help for both mother and baby. In some respects Erikson can be said to have done for the clinician what Piaget has done for teachers.

Studies of the global behaviour of children are not limited to the psychoanalytical approach, as is soon evident when we study the ethological approach.

Ethological contribution to child development (Barnett, 1962, 1967, 1973; Blurton Jones, 1972)

Ethology is the scientific study of animal behaviour and is said to be especially pertinent to an understanding of the manners of man and animals. The methods used by ethologists include observational techniques, experimental procedures and deductive reasoning. Studies have been centred upon birds, fish and animals because certain responses are more readily seen in some species than others, so that, by selecting an appropriate species to study, lessons can be learnt more easily. The faster rates of growth and maturation of some species mean that the full effects of experimental procedures are seen more quickly.

Ethologists have been criticized for assuming too readily that what they observe in artificial experimental procedures gives a true picture of what occurs naturally, and that the conclusions from animal studies can be transferred directly to humans. Despite these reservations, there is no doubt that ethology contributes much of value to our understanding of child development.

Ethological studies have revealed the complexity of development, and provided evidence to support both the maturational and the environmental hypotheses of development. On the one hand, the very complexity of many behavioural responses supports the maturational hypothesis, as it is difficult to conceive how such behaviours could otherwise occur. On the other hand, the variations of behaviour which ethologists have produced by environmental manipulation make it very clear that observed development results from the continual interaction of organism and environment.

Several ethological concepts are important in the study of child development. The term *instinct*, or *instinctive behaviour*, is applied to the complex stereotyped species-specific pattern of behaviour which is produced promptly and regularly by appropriate stimulation or *triggering*. These specific responses are elicited easily at certain periods, and less easily or not at all at other periods. The times of easy elicitation are called *sensitive periods*. Each specific pattern of behaviour has its own characteristic sensitive period (this term should not be confused with the term *critical period* which signifies an optimum period for learning responses).

Studies of the factors which lead to an ending of the sensitive periods have contributed to our understanding of the evolution of behaviour: aging and maturation (not synonymous, but related processes) are important influences, and with both there often is a change in the specific responses. Sometimes the sensitive period of a particular response is terminated by the appearance of other responses which interfere with it.

Learning also contributes to the extinction of the sensitive periods. The incorporation of a particular response into the learnt repertoire of an individual appears to inhibit the continued display of similar responses. When a response becomes incorporated into some other pattern of action, the instinctive aspect of the response ceases to be necessary, and it is both appropriate and desirable that it should fade away.

Closely linked with instinctive behaviour and the concept of sensitive periods is the phenomenon of *imprinting*. At an appropriate time an often rather bizarre, but nevertheless apparently biologically determined stimulus will trigger off a complex pattern of behaviour which may thereafter become well established. For example, a newly hatched duckling responds to the first moving object it perceives and automatically follows it, even if it is only a cardboard box pulled along the ground. And human babies a few weeks old show a smiling response to any disc-like object held before their eyes.

Opportunities to experience many stimuli and to exhibit a variety of responses appear to be essential for the development of all organisms. Childhood play is a rich source of both stimulation and opportunities for exercising responses. Ethologists have demonstrated experimentally the value of play for learning in many species, and also the long-range effects of deprivation of these opportunities. Observations such as those of Harlow upon the rearing of monkeys (Harlow and Suomi, 1971) have important lessons for all concerned with human development.

Ethology is particularly attractive for its contribution to a biological view of human development, but, like the other views of development, it is most useful when interpreted with the other views to produce an integrated picture of development.

An attempted synthesis

Several aspects of child development have been reviewed. There is much, however, which has not been included, such as the vast field of learning theory and the influence of different child-rearing practices, to mention just two topics. Nevertheless sufficient has been said to show the complexity of child development and the need for developmental paediatricians to have some insight into the various theories. But now some integration is necessary.

The contribution of these theories to our understanding of child development can be illustrated by considering a simple example – the response of a baby to a cube. Imagine a baby a few months old being placed in front of a table on which rests a small cube. Gesell's descriptions and our own observations tell us what happens. The baby looks around; he may give fleeting attention to the cube, but then becomes more interested in it as it is moved, or tapped on the table, and if the examiner is seen and speaks the infant is further encouraged. The baby reaches forward and grasps the cube in the palm of the hand. He may move his hand to bring the cube more clearly into his visual field. He may then move his hand and take the cube to his mouth. After a short while he drops the cube onto the table and appears to ignore it. A little later he accidentally touches the cube with his hand and responds as if this is his first encounter with the cube.

The baby's pattern of behaviour in such a situation is determined by his age, the stage of maturation of his nervous system, and by his previous experiences and what he has learnt from them. If he has had previous experience of manipulative exploration, he may then reach for the cube spontaneously without waiting for the additional stimuli of moving or tapping, or its demonstrated association with a familiar adult.

Reaching became a volitional act and the baby's principal means of tactile exploration because early arm movements, controlled by neurological reflexes such as the asymmetrical tonic neck reflex, produced random contact with objects.

Repetition of the action producing these tactile contacts led to its reinforcement and later incorporation as a voluntary act. In studying an infant's response to a cube, it is possible to see Piaget's stages of sensorimotor development. The fact that when the cube drops it leaves the child's awareness, and that when next he encounters it he comes upon it as an original experience, shows that the infant has not yet attained Piaget's stage of the awareness of the permanence of objects (which appears at about 8–9 months).

The infant reaches for the object with his arms, as these are the usual tactile exploratory limbs, but the essential drive here is for the infant to acquire knowledge of this external object; accordingly if his arms are paralysed or absent, he will attempt to reach by whatever means he has at his disposal – perhaps his leg, or his mouth, or even his eyes – and all these phenomena are shown by disabled children.

The mouthing of the cube is more than just another means of exploration. Erikson's views show how this oral exploration reassures the infant of the safety and security of the novel object in his environment.

The analysis of one simple situation, therefore, reveals much about the learning and development of the baby, and shows how the various views about development can be integrated.

Development occurs as the result of a biological drive which is characteristic of living organisms, and which follows a species-specific pattern. It begins by a succession of involuntary actions produced by the maturing nervous system. These actions are stimulated, or inhibited, or otherwise modified as a result of interaction with the environment and the individual's awareness and interpretation of the effects and results of this interaction, until they come under voluntary control.

Abnormalities of development arise in several ways: there may be slowing of the biological process so that the whole process of development follows its usual pattern, but at a much slower pace. This is *developmental lethargy*.

As a result of physical or sensory disabilities the individual may be unable to effect or appreciate the environmental interactions which provide the material for future learning, or the environmental opportunities may be lacking. Both these situations produce *developmental deprivation*.

On other occasions it seems as if the biological drive persists unaltered in strength, but the individual is unable to make use of and to learn from the interactions with the environment. In these situations it seems as if the persisting drive is easily diverted into bizarre and purposeless channels, producing *developmental non-assimilation* and *developmental distortion*.

Although much more needs to be learnt about child development, an appreciation of some of the theories does much to deepen one's understanding of this complex phenomenon. It also permits the creation of a working synthesis of the various views, and provides a basis for better understanding of both normal and deviant development.

References

Barnet, S. A. (1962) Lessons from animal behaviour for the clinician. *Clinics Dev. Med. 7.* London: Heinemann

Barnett, S. A. (1967) *Instinct and Intelligence*. London: MacGibbon and Kee

Barnett, S. A. (1973) Ethology and development. *Clinics Dev. Med. 47.* London: Heinemann

Blurton Jones, N. (1972) *Ethological Studies of Child Behaviour*. Cambridge: Cambridge University Press

Brearley, M. and Hitchfield, E. (1967) *A Teacher's Guide to Reading Piaget*. London: Routledge and Kegan Paul

Carmichael, L. (1926) The development of behaviour in vertebrates experimentally removed from the influence of external stimulation. *Psychol. Rev., 33*, 57

Dennis, W. (1943) The possibility of advancing and retarding the motor development of infants, *Psychol. Rev., 50*, 203

Erikson, E. H. (1967) *Childhood and Society*. London: Penguin Books

Flavell, J. H. (1963) *The Developmental Psychology of Jean Piaget*. Princeton, New Jersey: Van Nostrand

Gesell, A. (1948) *Studies in Child Development*. New York: Harper and Row

Gesell, A. (1966) *The First Five Years of Life*. London: Methuen

Gesell, A. and Amatruda, C. S. (1947) *Developmental Diagnosis*, 2nd edn. New York: Harper and Row

Gesell, A., Amatruda, C. S., Castner, B. M. and Thompson, H. (1930) *Biographies of Child Development*. London: Hamish Hamilton

Gesell, A. and Thompson, H. (1929) Learning and growth in identical twins; an experimental study by the method of co-twin control, *Genet. Psychol. Monogr., 6*, 1

Greenacre, P. (1944) Infant reactions to restraint. *Am. J. Orthopsychiat., 14*, 204

Harlow, H. F. and Suomi, S.J. (1971) Social recovery by isolation-reared monkeys, *Proc. Natl Acad. Sci. USA, 68*, 1534

Illingworth, R. S. (1958) Dissociation as a guide to developmental assessment, *Archs Dis. Childh., 33*, 118

McGraw, M. B. (1935) *Growth: A Study of Johnny and Jimmy*. New York: Appleton Century Crofts

Maier, H. W. (1969) *Three Theories of Child Development*. New York: Harper and Row

Winnicott, D. W. (1957) *The Child and the Outside World*. New York: Basic Books

Chapter 4

Integration of development: 'It all hangs together'

Children grow up and are adults before their parents know what is happening. They make tremendous advances with apparently little effort on their part or help from without. The magnitude of development, the apparent effortlessness with which it occurs and its strength are impressive features. Even in adverse circumstances children seem to have considerable resources for development. It could be the ease and inevitability of development which causes many people to take it for granted and so give it little attention or assistance.

A major process contributing to the apparent ease with which child development occurs is the integration of the various activities. Links develop between the various receptive channels; between the different expressive channels; and also between both of these groups. In addition, each new skill normally appears at the most appropriate time to make use of information coming in at that time; to carry out actions required at that time; and to prepare the way for the next stage of development. This sequential pattern may be distorted when there are delays and abnormalities of development, and a study of the effects produced by breakdowns in developmental integration seen in young disabled children provides considerable insight into the mechanisms of normal development.

Advantages of developmental integration

The many advantages of efficient developmental integration can be summarized as follows:

1. Increases in the scope of any one of the receptive channels by linking it with other receptive channels, and of the effectiveness of any action by links with other means of expressive response.
2. Increases in the potential for learning and for effective action.
3. Promotion of the smoothness of the developmental pattern.
4. Creation of a possibility of utilizing alternative means for acquiring information and carrying out actions. The possession of alternative means to achieve a particular goal is biologically most important, because if one route is blocked then compensatory mechanisms can be evoked. The importance of this is seen in the case of many disabled children.

Receptive integration

The full range of sensory-receptive links is shown in Figure 4.1. There are 10 dual combinations, all of which can be demonstrated to occur during the course of normal development. Some links become so established that they are accepted as one entity. For example, smell and taste are so intertwined that many people consider the two as one entity all the time. Some links, such as those between tactile sensation and smell and taste, are of little importance compared to others. The most important links are those between the auditory, visual and tactile sensory channels, as shown by the thicker lines in Figure 4.1. As these three modalities become associated in the course of normal development, any one, or a combination of two or all three, can be brought into use whenever necessary.

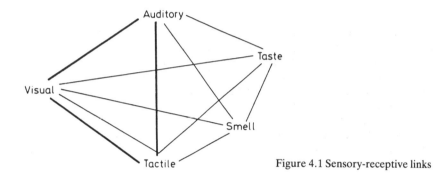

Figure 4.1 Sensory-receptive links

Infants are very receptive to all types of stimuli, but much of the information conveyed is new and strange to them. In order to be not just a passive recipient of stimuli infants have to apply considerable intellectual effort. At an early stage they show selective concentration upon one sensory channel and inhibition of other activities and interests. Visual, tactile and auditory preoccupation are terms which occur frequently in descriptions of child development between 6 and 12 months. Such preoccupation makes it difficult to examine infants. For example, failure to respond to sounds may not be due to deafness, but to intense visual or tactile preoccupation. Some normal infants seem to prefer one particular channel to the others and they present as predominantly visually, or auditorily, or tactilely interested babies. However, marked preference for one channel compared with the others should always lead to a careful check upon the intactness of the other channels.

Emergence from simple sensory preoccupation

Most infants show increasing ability to switch from one input channel to another. The succeeding steps can be summarized as follows:

(a) preoccupation with one sensory input at a time;
(b) increased flexibility to switch from channel to channel;
(c) comprehension of the nature of objects as perceived auditorily, visually and tactilely;

(d) ability to associate different sensory impressions about the same object received consecutively;

(e) ability to associate different sensory impressions about the same object received simultaneously;

(f) ability to receive simultaneous sensory impressions from different objects.

During the examination of infants it is useful to notice how they deal with multiple sensory stimuli. The observations give an indication of the maturity of development and can alert the developmental paediatrician to otherwise unsuspected abnormalities. It is highly probable that further study of this subject could lead to a fruitful means of early prediction of future potential.

Auditory-visual and auditory-tactile integration

In the early stages babies are aware of sounds but cannot locate them – they look vaguely in the general direction of the sound. With development their visual location becomes more precise until at about 9 months of age they can visually locate a sound source to within 5° – a good example of the development of auditory-visual integration. A baby who cannot make this auditory-visual link appears to be insecure as he searches for some tangible identification of the sounds.

Although in normal circumstances an auditory-tactile sensory link does not play a large part in development, it is invaluable for a blind child. Helping a blind baby to develop auditory-tactile integration can lead on to auditory language concepts and more effective interpretation of Braille through tactile sensation.

Visual-tactile integration

The integration of visual and tactile sensory functions is important for child development because even fully developed visual sensation does not provide all the available information about an observed object. It reveals size, shape and colour, but not weight, texture, consistency or temperature. These latter features can be learnt only by tactile exploration. So it is essential to have a visuo-tactile link if the maximum amount of information is to be learnt about the surrounding world. One remarkable case illustrated the limitations of experience which occur when tactile sensation is not available. The child concerned was severely affected by cerebral palsy and was completely unaware of the difference between sand and water. He had seen both flowing downwards from buckets as he watched children playing nearby in sandpits and pools, but because he had never had the tactile sensations, he was unaware of the dry grittiness of the sand and the smooth wetness of the water.

Visuo-tactile sensory links develop early in life as a result of action by the nervous system. The asymmetrical tonic neck reflex (ATNR) appears normally between 1 and 3 months of age. It extends the arm on the side to which the head is turned just at the time that visual fixation upon nearby objects is developing. The first tactile contact with the object the child is looking at is probably an accidental knocking of the object by the extended arm. After this accidental contact has occurred a few times, the infant may contrive for it to occur again until gradually a voluntary element is introduced into the action. From this beginning the infant rapidly builds up an ability to reach out, touch and even to take hold of the object he sees. Having served its purpose, the ATNR fades and so permits the next stage of development to occur.

Once the reflex ceases to dominate upper-limb posture, the hands can be brought together in the mid-line. This means that the infant can now look at an object, reach out towards it, take hold of it and then bring it into the mid-line closer to himself, so permitting a fuller examination of the object by mouthing, close visual inspection and, a little later, tactile exploration by the other hand. This is a neat example of developmental integration.

The linking of visuo-tactile sensations with appropriate motor actions leads to the acquisition of eye–hand co-ordination, which then develops rapidly and extensively from these early stages. Eye–hand co-ordination then becomes an essential part of the human motor skills and daily life activities. For example, a tennis player is able to see his opponent deliver a service, to judge the flight and speed of the ball, to place his racket in the correct position at the precise moment to ensure a good return shot, having glanced momentarily just before the shot to correct his positioning. And all this had to be done in about a tenth of a second! Such considerable skill develops out of developmental integration in the early months of life.

Expressive integration

The fact that sensory impressions are received through several different channels, and that it is advantageous to link these receptive functions, is easily understood and widely accepted. That a comparable situation exists on the expressive side is not so widely appreciated. At first sight there appear to be only two channels of response – motor actions and vocalizations – but these attributes are used so diversely that a very effective expressive repertoire is created (Figure 4.2).

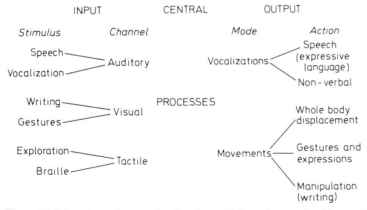

Figure 4.2 Receptive and expressive functions which can be associated by sensorimotor integration

From the expressive point of view, motor actions fall into three main categories, as follows:

1. Movement of the body, i.e. displacement, as when the child moves towards or away from a particular stimulus. The inhibition of movement is also important and can be considered in the same category. The ability to stand still is a valuable asset, for example, when listening.

2. Movements of various parts of the body, especially the face, eyes and arms, in ways which come to convey meaning. The value of gestures and facial expressions in everyday life is well appreciated by everyone.
3. Manipulation, which can take many forms; and, of course, modelling, drawing and writing are sophisticated forms of expression.

The other major channel of expression is through vocalization. Vocalization may be non-verbal or verbal. Non-verbal vocalizations such as shouting and crying and cooing can be very effective means of expression, often with a high emotional content. The great richness and effectiveness of verbal expressions needs little additional comment as it is so much part of all our lives.

The important aspect of development with respect to expressive functions is the acquisition of ability to select and control the responses. Some integration of actions is present from the beginning. The example of the young child who is frustrated and cross and who as a result cries, stamps his feet, waves his arms, runs away and crossly denounces everyone is familiar to all. As development occurs, control over the integrated actions is achieved and responses are modified accordingly.

Receptive–expressive integration

Essential to child development are the integrative links which occur between receptive and expressive functions. The range of these functions is shown in Figure 4.2. The central neurological processes play an all-important role in creating and maintaining this integration.

Developmental paediatricians must consider the links between receptive and expressive functions with regard to both their contributions to the child's development and the effects of their absence.

Auditory-vocal integration

Children receive, by the auditory channel, many sounds which include non-verbal and verbal vocalizations. The range of their own vocalizations depends upon the frequency, richness and clarity of the input received from others and when such input is missing, as in the case of a severely deprived child or a deaf child, the expressive side does not develop. The normal pattern is for children to understand what they hear before they are able to reproduce it themselves. If the imperfect utterances of a young child are played back to him, he is usually irritated because he is used to hearing and understanding much clearer speech than he can produce himself. The internal auditory feedback mechanism constantly monitors the vocal expressions from an early age and this monitoring ensures that what is expressed is what was intended to be expressed. A delay in auditory feedback of even less than a second produces confusion and frustration and inhibits the free flow of expressive language.

Auditory-motor integration

Auditory reception is enhanced by motor activity. The ability to turn the head helps to locate sounds; to be able to move to the source of sounds and to produce sounds by using the hands for clapping and plucking a musical instrument increase the awareness of, and interest in, sounds. To be able to stop movement helps the child to concentrate on 'listening'. However, if the movements do not correspond with the requirements of auditory reception, then difficulties arise and development is disrupted. For example, young children receive auditory stimuli at 'knee level' as they sit on their mother's lap and she speaks to them with her mouth only a few inches from the child's ear. When the child can slip off the knee and crawl or walk across the room, he immediately extends the distance between himself and his mother's voice. If he is ready for this move, he retains auditory awareness and receptivity at the greater distance, but if he is not ready he moves out of the zone of verbal stimulation and an arrest occurs in language development. This phenomenon is seen in some mobile, mentally handicapped children, as shown in Figure 4.3.

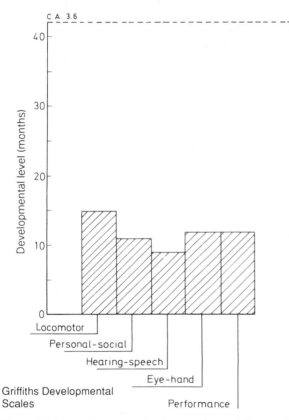

Figure 4.3 Arrest of language development in a mobile mentally handicapped child aged 3 years 6 months

Normally mobility occurs at just the right stage, and the greater number of personal contacts and opportunities for exploration enjoyed by the mobile child increases his vocabulary and language. In this respect motor activity and auditory reception work together to promote development. In contrast a child who cannot move about has to wait until others come near for him to hear what they say and for them to hear what he says. This can be a very stultifying experience and adversely affects the child's development.

Visual-vocal integration

Reading aloud is a ready example of visual-vocal integration. The visual input is interpreted centrally, formulated into auditory language and then expressed vocally. Vocalizations express reactions to visual events such as a gasp of delight at a particularly beautiful scene. Verbal ability is used to describe what is seen, and this skill can be used to communicate with others and to direct one's own actions. In these ways visual-vocal integration plays a frequent and important role in development and failure of this integration leads to serious consequences, most important perhaps being various reading disabilities.

Visual-motor integration

Visual reception and perception provide information about the size, shape and colour of objects, their position and relationship with one another, and their movements. This applies to both external objects and to one's own body. Motor activities enable one to move about oneself and also to move other objects. This reinforces visual perception and leads to the development of awareness of spatial dimensions, movement and speed. The ability to move oneself, whether this be of the whole body or a fine manipulative movement, and the ability to move other things, enhance visual perception and learning, and without these motor experiences development suffers. In a widely known experiment described by Held and Hein (1963), two kittens were placed at either end of a roundabout arm. One was harnessed to the roundabout and provided the motor activity to turn it. The other was a passive passenger positioned at the end of the roundabout arm. The active kitten of each experimental pair responded better than the passive kitten in subsequent tests of motor ability, indicating that self-produced movement with concurrent visual feedback is necessary for the development of visually guided behaviour.

The integration of visual reception with motor activity in the development of eye–hand co-ordination has been described already.

Tactile-vocal integration

Tactile sensations can provoke vocalizations, especially if they are particularly extreme. The information obtained by tactile exploration is enhanced by verbal labelling and description. Braille reading is an example of sophisticated tactile information being interpreted and understood and then reproduced as expressive language.

Tactile-motor integration

Motor activities increase the range and scope of tactile exploration. Children who do not possess arms utilize whatever means they have to obtain tactile information. This might be by using their feet or their mouth. Tactile sensations frequently provide the information for motor action. For example, touching a hot plate leads to rapid withdrawal of the hand.

Conclusion

The associations described above are important for child development and can assume great importance in certain circumstances. As one studies child development, it is necessary to examine each function and to consider whether or not attempts are being made to integrate this with other functions; whether this integration is proceeding appropriately and adequately; whether it is so efficient that it has been internalized; or so deficient that problems are arising and special help is needed. Much of the developmental guidance programmes for handicapped children is concerned with stimulation of the associative processes.

References
Held, R. and Hein, A. (1963) Movement-producing stimulation in the development of visually guided behaviour. *J. Comp. Physiol. Psychol.*, **56**, 872

Part II

Normal development

Chapter 5

The neonate and reflex activity in infancy

Human development requires many years to reach completion. Life begins with the union of two minute cells which then quickly multiply and differentiate so that at birth some 40 weeks later the baby already weighs about 3.5 kg (7.7 lb), and is a complex organism (Figure 5.1).

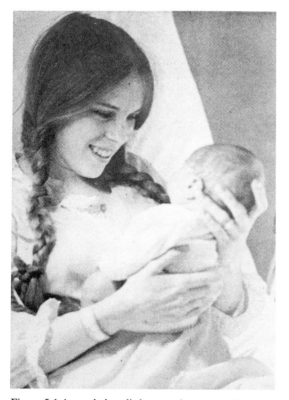

Figure 5.1 A new baby – little more than a twentieth the size of the mother

In one respect the neonate is reasonably well equipped biologically for survival outside the uterus. Basic bodily functions such as circulation, respiration, digestion, elimination, homeostasis and temperature regulation are well developed. In other respects the neonate is quite immature. Sensory perception is not fully developed, and it takes a long time for him to acquire mobility and manipulative skills and to learn to utilize all his potential abilities.

Flexion dominates the neonate's postures. When he is picked up and laid in a prone position, the head turns sideways as a result of a protective reflex which prevents suffocation, the arms are flexed, and the legs are flexed and drawn up under the abdomen so that the pelvis is raised (Figure 5.2). Some movements of the limbs and trunk occur in this position, but they occur more freely in the supine position, because the limbs are less restricted. There is very little control at this stage and the head flops downwards when the baby is lifted into ventral suspension (i.e. supported in a prone position with a hand under the abdomen), or into a sitting posture.

The neonate shows awareness of both auditory and visual stimuli by quietening if the stimuli are tolerable, or by blinking, grimacing, startling and crying if they are stronger.

The neonate exhibits a number of reflexes in which a relatively minor stimulus suffices to trigger off an almost instantaneous stereotyped response. These primary

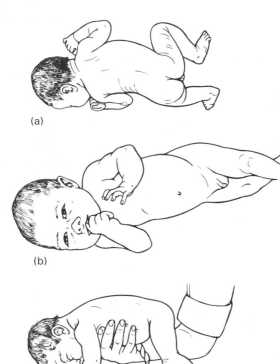

(a)

(b)

(c)

Figure 5.2 The neonate: (a) prone; (b) supine; (c) ventral suspension

reflexes demonstrate the activity of the neonate's central nervous system and they provide the basis for later motor development.

The nervous system of a newly born baby is well developed and capable of complex activities. This is shown, for example, by the facts that the neurological control of such a vital function as breathing is well established, and that there are many reflex responses which can be obtained by appropriate stimulation. But this is not the final state and further development of the nervous system occurs rapidly during the early years.

A reflex action consists of a prompt, stereotyped and often very considerable response to a specific and often quite minor stimulus. There is no opportunity for variation or choice of action.

As the nervous system develops, many of the early reflexes are inhibited, and others are modified and incorporated into more complex actions. These changes are necessary because continued activity of the early reflexes would interfere with the development of other actions, an effect which is seen in some neurologically disabled children.

The pattern of reflexes reflects the phylogenetic evolution of the nervous system. Many of the reflexes are evident in other species. For example, the trunk-righting reflexes are also shown by quadrupeds. Some reflexes are considered to be the persisting remnants of vitally important ones in the past. For example, the grasp reflex would serve an essential survival function when it was necessary for the animal infant to be able to cling to the mother's fur. Other reflexes are unique to man, especially those concerned with the attainment and maintenance of the upright posture.

Our understanding of reflex activity in the infant comes from several sources, including neurophysiological experimental studies and observations of the evolution of reflex activity in both normal and abnormal babies. Sherrington (1898), Magnus and de Kleijn (1930), Magnus (1961) and Rademaker (l961) were concerned with identifying the areas and pathways within the brain used by the various reflexes, and they showed, among many other things, the important role of the labyrinth for the maintenance of the upright posture and balance. Peiper (1961) was convinced of the importance of the neurophysiological approach in understanding cerebral function in infancy and childhood, and reference to his work is recommended to all who seek to understand reflex activity in early life. Other useful references in this connection are to Thomas, Chesni and Dargassies (1960), Paine and Opie (1966) and Milani Comparetti and Gidoni (1967).

Clinical and developmental significance of reflexes

Some of the many reflexes which have been described are of only passing interest and curiosity, whereas others are more important because they provide useful diagnostic signs; they influence the child's development; and they can be used therapeutically.

Those reflexes which are of diagnostic value indicate abnormality by their weakness, absence, excessive strength or persistence to an inappropriate age. For example, the Moro reflex is a particularly useful diagnostic reflex. It is present so consistently and is so easily elicitable in the newborn period that any variation from the fully normal response at this time is a reliable indication of probable abnormality, and its persistence after 6 months of age also indicates abnormality.

The most interesting reflexes are those which influence development. For example, the asymmetrical tonic neck reflex is normally most evident at 2–3 months of age when it appears to prepare the way for the integration of head turning, visual fixation and reaching, and so is probably fundamental to the establishment of visually directed reaching and eye–hand co-ordination. That reflex affects development favourably. An example of a reflex which impedes development as a result of its abnormal persistence is seen with respect to the grasp reflex. Manipulative skill is one of man's great assets which requires individual finger action and release, but these become possible only as the grasp reflex wanes and its persistence delays the acquisition of such skill.

Some reflexes are utilized in therapeutic programmes for children with cerebral palsy. For example, tactile stimulation in certain areas is used to promote reflex muscle contractions and movements.

Qualifying definitions

The simplest reflex consists of a prompt, but brief stereotyped response to an appropriate stimulus. Many of the reflexes elicited in a clinical examination are of this nature. Others are more complex. Some show a persistence of the response as long as the stimulus lasts – this is called a *tonic* effect. Some reflexes, especially those concerned with posture and movement, trigger off a series of *chain responses* which may lead to some form of effective action. Very forceful reflexes which cannot be resisted and overcome are said to be *obligatory*. An obligatory response is usually abnormal.

Changes with age

The pattern of reflex activity changes with age. Some activity can be seen quite early in fetal life. Thereafter it increases rapidly both in intensity and complexity. The study of the appearance and evolution of reflex activity from fetal life and infancy onwards is a fascinating exercise which provides much insight into the elaboration of the nervous system. The reflexes fade after serving their purpose or as they are superseded by others, but they seldom disappear entirely. Normally they persist throughout life without our being aware of them. For example, the continued maintenance of our posture and movement against gravity is possible only as a result of the continued action of the reflex postural mechanisms, and we only become aware of this when control is lost. Reflexes sometimes reappear following cerebral catastrophe in later life.

Production by several stimuli

In a pure reflex a specific stimulus is followed by a stereotyped and predictable response. The afferent stimulus may be auditory, visual, tactile (especially touch, pressure and pain), labyrinthine or kinaesthetic. Sometimes different stimuli give rise to similar responses. This phenomenon is valuable biologically because it ensures that if one method of elicitation fails others will still produce the appropriate responses. For example, head-righting upon the body may occur as the result of kinaesthetic stimulation from the neck, optic stimulation and labyrinthine stimulation. When several different stimuli can produce a particular reflex response their relative importance varies, and each may predominate at different stages of development.

Terminology confusion

Unnecessary confusion is produced when the same response is described as different reflexes according to the way it is produced. For example, pressure upon the sole of an infant's foot causes the leg to extend. The essential stimulus comes from the sole of the foot and the response consists of extension of the leg. When this reflex is elicited by holding the infant upright and allowing the sole of the foot to contact a flat surface, the response constitutes a useful anti-gravity supporting reaction and it is often given this name. The reflex can also be demonstrated with

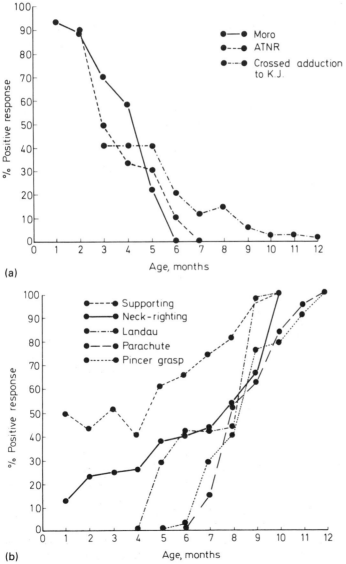

(a)

(b)

Figure 5.3 Some primary reflexes which (a) disappear and some secondary reflexes which (b) appear during the first year (After Paine and Opie, 1966)

the child lying down. The sole of the foot is touched by the examiner's hand and as this hand is withdrawn the leg extends as if following the stimulating hand. This is called the magnet reflex. These are not different reflexes; the magnet reflex is basically identical with the supporting reaction.

Classification

Reflexes may be grouped in several ways. They may be grouped according to their function. Some are protective and have a survival value for the infant; others promote appropriate orientation, as for feeding (e.g. rooting reflex) and use of the sensory organs; and others promote postural support and balance.

Reflexes may be grouped according to their time of appearance – the primary reflexes are present at birth and then fade to be replaced by secondary reflexes. Figure 5.3 shows several primary reflexes which disappear during the first year and other secondary reflexes which appear in the second 6 months of the first year.

Reflexes may also be grouped according to the method of elicitation, or by the part of the body taking part in the reflex.

The better known and more important reflexes are described below. They are grouped according to the type of stimulus required for their initiation.

Reflex responses to light touch

Light touch produces a variety of reflex responses depending upon the area stimulated and the age of the individual. The motor responses are most marked in the early months of life.

Grasp reflex: palmar and plantar
Light touch of the palm or sole produces reflex flexion of the fingers or toes. The most effective way to elicit the reflex is to slide the stimulating object such as a finger or pencil across the palm or sole from the lateral border. Prechtl (1953) described the beautiful neurological organization of the palmar grasp reflex in which finger flexion follows a definite sequence: mid–ring–little–index–thumb (Figure 5.4).

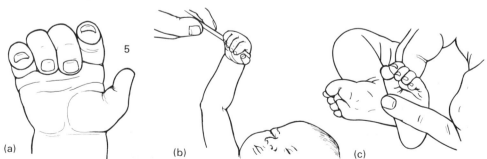

Figure 5.4 The grasp reflex: (a) sequence of finger flexion; (b) tonic component of the palmar grasp reflex; (c) plantar grasp reflex

Chain responses follow the initial reflex producing two further stages which are seen best in the palmar reflex. The first follows initial flexion of the digits and consists of tensing of the flexed muscles to produce a strong grasp. A strong tonic component at this stage of the reflex ensures maintenance of the grasp as long as the stimulus persists. The second stage occurs when traction is exerted by the stimulating finger or pencil. There follows a progressive contraction of the arm muscles which is sometimes so strong that the baby can be lifted from the examination couch. The palmar and plantar grasp reflexes are easily demonstrable in the neonate, but then fade rapidly and are seldom seen after 4 or 5 months of age.

Phylogenetically the reflex is suggested to have had survival value by enabling the infant to cling to the mother's fur.

Placing reflex (Figure 5.5)

Stimulation of the dorsum of the foot of the neonate produces flexion of the same leg. Probably the easiest way to show this, and the method used in clinical examination, is to hold the infant upright and to let the dorsum of the foot touch the lower side of the edge of the table. The infant flexes the leg and appears to do so in order to place the foot on the table. This reflex is readily demonstrable in the newborn and persistent failure to elicit it at this stage is thought to indicate neurological abnormality. It fades rapidly in the early months.

Rooting reflex

Light touch of the cheek or stimulation of the edge of the mouth results in turning of the head in the direction of the stimulus and simultaneous opening of the mouth and extension of the tongue (Figure 5.6). It is sometimes called the cardinal points

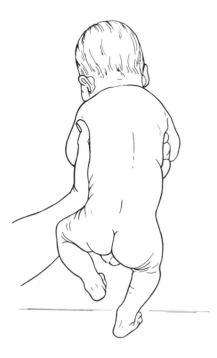

Figure 5.5 The placing reflex (the left leg is flexed after the dorsum of the foot touched the table edge – the right leg is about to be stimulated in the same way)

reflex because it is elicited by stimulation of all four quadrants around the mouth. The reflex appears to have an adaptive and survival function. Utilization of the reflex during feeding ensures that the infant takes the nipple well into its widely opened mouth and so avoids painful pressure upon the end. Undue haste over breast feeding or other faulty techniques which prevent use of this reflex lead to incomplete acceptance of the nipple into the infant's mouth and cause discomfort. The reflex is demonstrable in the newborn period and then fades during the early months. I have found it valuable to use this reflex to obtain an indication of the infant's alertness by noting its ease of elicitation (Holt, 1972).

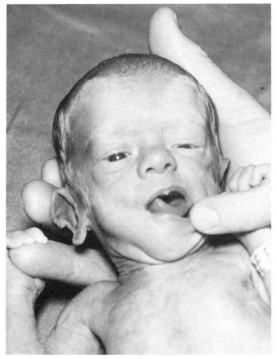

Figure 5.6 Elicitation of the rooting (cardinal points) reflex

Reflex responses to pressure and pain

Although some of the responses to pressure serve a constructive and functional role (such as the support reaction), the majority have a protective and survival value (e.g. the withdrawal response). Many of these responses are so well ingrained that only the most profound cerebral depression inhibits them; for example, the persistent absence of Galant's response in the neonatal period indicates severe disturbance and a poor prognosis.

Galant's reflex (Figure 5.7)
Firm sharp stimulation alongside the spine with the finger nails or a pin produces contraction of the underlying muscles and curving of the back. This response is

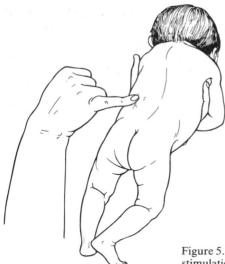

Figure 5.7 Galant's reflex (trunk incurvation). Following stimulation, the back is arched concave to the stimulating finger

readily seen when the infant is held upright and the trunk movement is unrestricted while the stimulus is applied. It is best seen in the neonatal period and thereafter gradually fades.

Withdrawal reflex (Figure 5.8)
A pinprick or other sharp painful stimulus results in flexion and withdrawal of the stimulated limb. This is best seen in the leg when the sole of the foot is stimulated in this way. The protective value of the reflex is obvious.

(a)

(b)

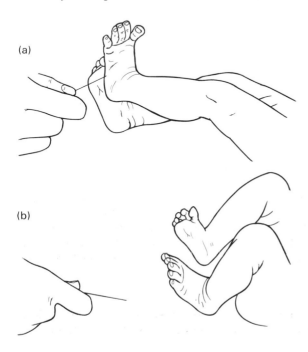

Figure 5.8 The withdrawal reflex: (a) stimulation; (b) response

Crossed extension reflex (Figure 5.9)

If the leg is kept extended at the knee while the sole of the foot is stimulated by firm strokes with a finger or other firm object, the opposite leg flexes and then extends. Because the extension phase is associated with some adduction at the hip, an impression is obtained of the moving leg crossing the stimulated one as if to push away the stimulating hand. This reflex is present in the neonate and even in the premature baby. Brett (1965) uses the reflex when determining the maturity of the newborn. The reflex gradually fades during the first year, but it is difficult to ascribe a precise time after which it is no longer seen. I have been impressed by the diagnostic value of this reflex, having found it to be present at 1 year of age as the only clue to diagnosis in several babies who later showed a well-developed picture of cerebral palsy.

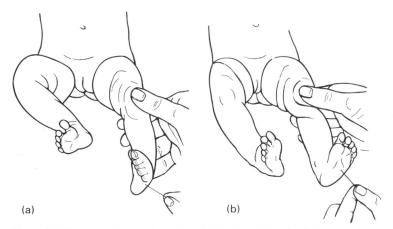

(a)   (b)

Figure 5.9 The crossed extension reflex: (a) flexion of right leg following stimulation of sole of the left foot, then (b) extension of the right leg

Babinski (plantar) reflex (Holt, 1961) (Figure 5.10)

This reflex is one of the fundamental signs of classical neurology. The stimulus consists of a firm painful stroke along the lateral border of the sole from heel to toe. The response consists of movement (flexion or extension) of the big toe and sometimes movement (fanning) of the other toes. Techniques have been described to elicit the response by stimulating other areas (e.g. stroking the lateral border of the dorsum of the foot, squeezing the calf, or running the fingers along the anterior border of the tibia). These manoeuvres are most effective when the reflex is pathologically exaggerated.

   The reflex is present throughout life. In the first year or two the surface area from which stimuli are effective is quite extensive. Thereafter it shrinks until the lateral side of the sole is the principal area from which a response can be obtained. The motor response is similarly widespread at first, so that movement of all the toes is noticeable, and extension of the big toe usually predominates over the weaker flexion movement. After this age, however, the motor response becomes more controlled and restricted.

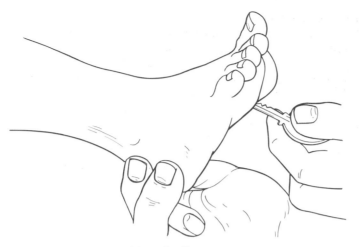

Figure 5.10 The Babinski (plantar) reflex

The extensors of the big toe do not appear to be stimulated, so flexion of the big toe becomes the normal response. It is probable that progressive reduction of both the area of effective stimulation and the changes in the motor response reflect increasing neurological maturation. After two or three years of age, extension of the big toe is abnormal and usually indicates a lesion of the pyramidal tract. This reflex is most useful diagnostically, and great reliance is placed upon it in neurological examinations.

Magnet (traction) reflex (Figure 5.11)
Steady firm pressure is applied to the sole of the foot or to the palm of the hand with the limb flexed, and is then gently withdrawn to be followed by extension of the limb as if being drawn forwards by a magnet. This reflex is demonstrable in the early months.

Babkin reflex
The stimulus for this reflex consists of deep pressure applied simultaneously to the palms of both hands while the infant is in an appropriate position, ideally supine. The stimulus is followed by flexion or forward bowing of the head, opening of the mouth and closing of the eyes. The reflex can be demonstrated in the newborn, thus showing a hand–mouth neurological link even at that early stage. It fades rapidly, and normally cannot be elicited after 4 months of age. Elicitation of the reflex after this age indicates a cerebral lesion.

Stepping reflex (Figure 5.12)
Pressure upon the sole of the foot of the neonate causes first flexion then extension of the leg. As this occurs on alternate sides, an impression is created of automatic stepping. It is not true walking, however, because there is no trunk support or pelvic stability – this is acquired through the support reflex which develops later. MacKeith (1964) showed very neatly that head position affected the ease of elicitation, strength and duration of this reflex. The stepping reflex should

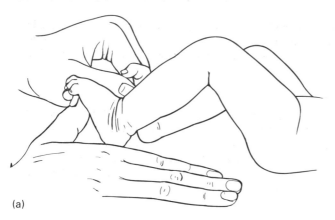

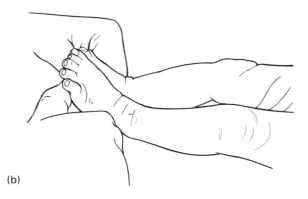

(a)

(b)

Figure 5.11 The magnet reflex: (a) stimulation; (b) response

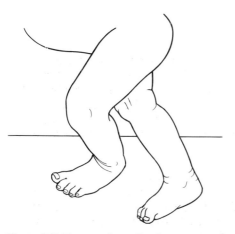

Figure 5.12 The stepping reflex (contact of the sole with the table top produces flexion of the leg and alternate stepping)

disappear by 6 months of age. This reflex sometimes persists for many years in children with cerebral palsy, and parents think that their child must be near to walking, little realizing that he is merely demonstrating the persistence of a primitive reflex.

Support reflex (legs) (Figure 5.13)

The similarity of this reflex to the magnet reflex was mentioned earlier. When an infant is held vertically and the soles of the feet allowed to come into contact with a table or floor, the pressure on the soles causes reflex extension of the legs. A chain response producing secondary stiffening of the legs follows the initial reaction and makes the legs strong supporting pillars. This complex reflex is important for the development of the upright posture and locomotion.

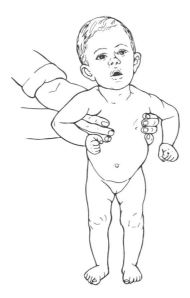

Figure 5.13 The support reflex of lower limbs

The reflex is elicited with difficulty in the early months and even when it is obtained it lasts only a few brief moments. It gradually becomes more evident as the stepping reflex fades, and by 6 months of age it should be obtained readily and persist for several minutes. Failure of this reflex to appear at the right time delays locomotor development. Persistence long after it has served its purpose is a sign of neurological abnormality, and also produces characteristic abnormal gait patterns.

Support reflex (arms) (Figure 5.14)

A support reflex appears in the arms several months later than the similar reflex in the legs. As the body is tilted forwards or sideways, extension of the arms occurs. Contact of the palms of the open hands with a firm surface then provides the stimulus for tensing of the arm muscles. Visual and labyrinthine righting reflexes are responsible for the early part of the reflex and support follows pressure stimulus on the palms.

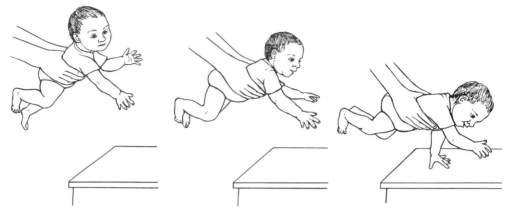

Figure 5.14 The support reflex of upper limbs

Reflex responses to kinaesthetic stimuli

Many reflex responses originate from stimuli from the tendons, muscles and joints. Most of them are important in the maintenance of posture and orientation of the body in space.

Tendon reflexes

These are simple monosynaptic spinal reflexes which are elicited by a sudden stretch of a muscle tendon such as occurs when the tendon is tapped. They are present throughout life and are most useful diagnostically for the detection of upper motor neurone lesions (exaggerated response); myopathic conditions (depressed or absent response); and localization of segmental lesions of the cord. The cord levels served by the various tendon reflexes are shown in Table 5.1.

Table 5.1 Spinal cord levels of the tendon reflexes

Reflex	Cord level
Biceps (elbow)	C5,6
Brachioradialis	C5,6
Triceps	C6,8
Long finger flexors	C6–T1
Abductors	L2,4
Quadriceps (knee)	L2,4
Gastrocnemius–soleus (ankle)	S1,2

C, cervical; T, thoracic; L, lumbar; S, sacral.

Eye righting (doll's eye) reflex (Figure 5.15)

Passive turning of the head of the newborn leaves the eyes 'behind' and a distinct time lag occurs before the eyes move to a new position in keeping with the head position. Within a week or two of birth, this doll's eye phenomenon has

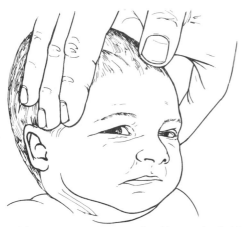

Figure 5.15 The doll's eye reflex (the eyes lag behind as the head rotates)

disappeared as a result of an eye righting reflex. Failure of this reflex to appear, i.e. persistence of the doll's eye phenomenon, indicates a cerebral lesion. Although this reflex is listed here with the reflex responses to kinaesthetic stimuli, it is probable that the labyrinths also have a major influence on the reflex (Kestenbaum, 1930).

Moro reflex (Figure 5.16)
This is one of the best known and most useful of all the neonatal reflexes. The afferent stimulus is a sudden movement of the head on the shoulders. It can be produced in several ways. One way is to allow the head to drop about 25 mm (1 in) into the palm of the hand; another way is to raise the supine baby a short way from the couch by pulling upon the hands and then releasing them suddenly. The response consists of wide abduction of the arms and opening of the hands. Within moments the arms come together again simulating an embrace. The response often includes tensing of the back muscles, flexion of the legs and crying. The response should be symmetrical; asymmetry indicates a central or peripheral nervous system lesion, or injury to the bones or muscles of the defective arm. Failure of the arms to move freely and of the hands to open fully indicates hypertonia, and feebleness of response occurs with hypotonia and prematurity. The reflex is present at birth. Its persistent absence or asymmetry in a newborn should cause considerable concern. It fades rapidly and is not normally elicitable after 6 months of age.

Asymmetrical tonic neck reflex (ATNR) (Figure 5.17)
The stimulus which initiates this reflex consists of sideways turning of the head, either passively or actively. The response consists of extension of the arm on the side to which the head turns and flexion of the opposite arm. Similar movements occur in the legs. The precise age at which this reflex appears continues to be the subject of controversy; some deny that it is present in the neonatal period, whereas others think that it can be produced at that early stage. It is certainly not frequently seen nor easily elicited at that time, and it is most evident between 2 and 3 months of age.

This reflex would seem to play an important role in visuomotor development. It is present during the time that visual fixation upon nearby objects is developing and it seems that the nervous system is making sure that the appropriate arm stretches

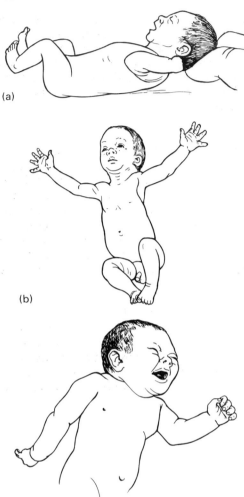

(a)

(b)

(c)

Figure 5.16 The Moro reflex: (a) one method of elicitation; (b) normal response; (c) asymmetrical response due to Erb's palsy

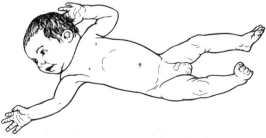

Figure 5.17 The asymmetrical tonic neck reflex

out towards visualized objects. As the hand touches the object the seeds are sown of awareness of distance ('at arm's length') and eye–hand co-ordination.

The reflex fades rapidly and is not normally seen after 6 months of age. Persistence of the ATNR is the most frequently observed abnormality of the infantile reflexes in infants with neurological lesions (Paine, 1964). Its persistence, usually in an exaggeratedly strong form, is a clear indication of abnormality of the nervous system and greatly disrupts development.

Symmetrical tonic neck reflex

Experimental observations of animals have shown that flexion and extension of the head can profoundly influence the posture of the animal. The response has been linked with their feeding needs and habits. When the reflex is strong in an experimental dog, for example, flexion of the head causes flexion of the fore limbs and extension of the hind limbs, just as if the animal was bending the head forward in order to take food; whereas extension of the head produces extension of the fore limbs and flexion of the hind limbs, just as if the animal was preparing to take a tasty morsel held above him. This reflex is not normally easily seen or elicited in normal infants, but may be seen in exaggerated form in some children with cerebral palsy.

Head–body and body–head righting reflexes (Figure 5.18)

As mentioned earlier, various stimuli may produce the same response. Orientation of the head in relation to the body and vice versa is so important that it is not surprising that it is produced by several righting reflexes. Some of them arise from kinaesthetic stimulation of the muscles and joints of the neck. As the head is turned, the trunk realigns itself so as to remain in normal relationship to the head.

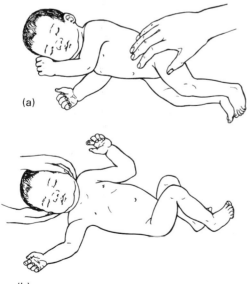

(a)

(b)

Figure 5.18 (a) Head righting reflex (rotation of the trunk is followed by righting of the head). (b) Body righting reflex (rotation of the head is followed by righting of the trunk)

Similarly, turning of the trunk is followed by reorientation of head position. These righting reflexes are present early in life, and during the second half of the first year of life they reinforce the action of the visual and labyrinthine righting reflexes. A clear understanding of the righting reflexes is necessary for the treatment of young children with central neurological disorders. For example, in the case of a child who cannot roll sideways it is necessary to study these reflexes to know whether it is therapeutically better to rotate the head and have the trunk follow or vice versa.

Reflex responses to visual and auditory stimuli

As our visual and auditory senses are able to receive stimuli from a distance, they are well equipped to act as warning mechanisms. Consequently many of the reflexes produced by visual and auditory stimuli have a protective and survival value.

Blink reflex
A bright light suddenly shone into the eyes, a puff of air upon the sensitive cornea or a sudden loud noise produce immediate blinking of the eyes. There may be associated tensing of the neck muscles and turning of the head away from the stimulus, and grimacing and crying. These reflexes are easily seen in the neonate in whom the responses are well marked and widespread. They continue to be present throughout life.

Visual righting reflex (Figure 5.19)
Once some visual awareness of orientation has developed, infants do not readily tolerate distorted views and reflexly attempt to right their head position in order to correct the view. This visual righting reflex develops in close association with the labyrinthine righting reflexes.

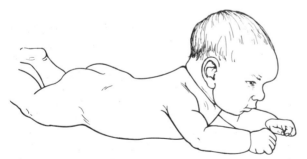

Figure 5.19 Head extension due to labyrinthine head righting reflex reinforced by visual righting reflex

Auditory orientating reflexes (Figure 5.20)
A sudden noise, especially if it is loud and unpleasant, may produce the blink reflex as described above, or the infant may remain still and show increased alertness. Quieter sounds usually cause reflex eye and head turning to the side of the sound, as if to locate it. This auditory orientation reflex is seen first clearly about 4 months of age. Thereafter head turning towards sound stimuli becomes more complex, and

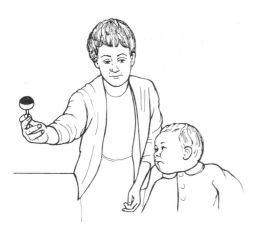

Figure 5.20 Head turning to auditory stimulus

the accuracy of localization increases rapidly until by 9–10 months the sound source is located directly and promptly within about 5° (Murphy, 1962). These reflex responses are made use of in tests of infants for hearing loss. The pattern of the localization responses also indicates the level of neurological maturity.

Reflex response to labyrinthine stimuli

The attainment and maintenance of upright postures against gravity are essential requirements for the successful motor development of the human infant. The labyrinths are the most important organs concerned with the development of anti-gravity postures and balance. Movement of the head in any dimension stimulates some part of the labyrinths and, after the early weeks, produces appropriate responses.

Labyrinthine head righting
Once this reflex has developed, the infant's head is always moved into a position in which the vertex is uppermost and the mouth horizontal whatever the position of the child. Thus, if the infant is held by the feet with the trunk and head downwards, the head will be extended backwards in order to get it upright against gravity. Similarly, if the infant is held in ventral suspension, i.e. horizontally with a hand supporting the trunk, the head will be extended to achieve an upright posture. The response elicited in this latter position has been described as the Landau reflex.

Labyrinthine head righting is not present at birth (Figure 5.21), but develops during the early months. Its influence is clearly seen in the progressive ease with which the infant raises his head in the prone position. In humans, head righting responses also occur in response to visual stimuli, so that when observing the motor development of infants it is difficult to know the relative contributions made by these two head righting mechanisms. Those children who fail to develop any head righting ability at all, such as some children with cerebral palsy, are very disabled in consequence.

The development of head righting and of the ability to control the head position irrespective of gravity opens up great possibilities for further motor development. A series of chain reactions ensue as various reflexes influence the body position and

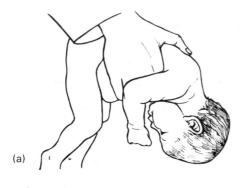

(a)

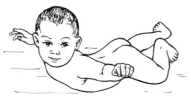

(b)

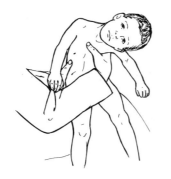

(c)

Figure 5.21 Head righting: (a) absence in neonate; (b) ease of head raising in prone position at 8 months; (c) absence in child with cerebral palsy

the attitudes and movements of the limbs. For example, once an infant can raise his head in the prone position the way is open for him to crawl. The sequence is as follows:

Head righting – increases in strength and extent until shoulders are raised – this facilitates forward movement of arms – support reflex of arms then enables chest to be raised – this facilitates raising of pelvis – leads to drawing up of knees and then support reflex enables pelvis to be raised – as security of support increases, limbs can be freed in succession to develop an alternating reciprocal movement – crawling is achieved.

Tonic labyrinthine reflexes
The labyrinths are thought to exert a tonic influence upon the distribution of muscle tone throughout the body, and to control the balance between the extensor and flexor muscles. It is very difficult to isolate and study these effects in normal infants, but the effects of disturbances of these tonic reflexes are very obvious in neurologically damaged infants, many of whom exhibit dystonic syndromes.

References

Brett, E. M. (1965) The estimation of foetal maturity by the neurological examination of the neonate. *Clinics Dev. Med. 19.* London: Heinemann

Holt, K. S. (1961) The plantar response in infants and children. *Cerebr. Palsy Bull.,* **3,** 449

Holt, K. S. (1972). Neurological examination of the newborn. *Hosp. Med. NY,* **8,** 86

Kestenbaum, A. (1930) Zur Entwickling der Angenbewagungen und des Optokinetishen Nystagmus. *Archs Ophth.,* **124,** 113

MacKeith, R. C. (1964) The primary walking response and its facilitation by passive extension of the head. *Acta Paediat.,* **17,** suppl. 6

Magnus, R. (1961) Korperstellung. In *Cerebral Function in Infancy and Childhood* (ed. A. Peiper). London: Pitman Medical

Magnus, R. and de Kleijn, A. (1930) Korperstellung, Gleichgewicht und Bewegung bei Saugern. Haltung und Stellung bei Saugern. *Handb. Physiol.,* **15,** 1, 29 and 55

Milani Comparetti, A. and Gidoni, E. A. (1967) Routine developmental examination in normal and retarded children. *Devl. Med. Child Neurol.,* **9,** 631

Murphy, K. P. (1962) Ascertainment of deafness in children. *Panorama,* Dec. 3. Reading: Linco Acoustics Ltd

Paine, R. (1964). The evolution of infantile postural reflexes in the presence of chronic syndromes. *Devl. Med. Child Neurol.,* **6,** 345

Paine, R. S. and Opie, T. E. (1966). Neurological examination of children. *Clinics Dev. Med. 20/21.* London: Heinemann

Peiper, A. (1961) *Cerebral Function in Infancy and Childhood.* London: Pitman Medical

Prechtl, H. F. R. (1953) *Umschau,* **53,** 656

Rademaker, G. G. J. (1961) Das Stehen. In *Cerebral Function in Infancy and Childhood* (ed. A. Peiper). London: Pitman Medical

Sherrington, C. S. (1898) Decerebrate rigidity and reflex coordination of movements. *J. Physiol.,* **22,** 319

Thomas, A., Chesni, J. and Dargassies, S. Saint-Anne (1960) The neurological examination of the infant. *Little Club Clinics 1.* London: Heinemann

Chapter 6

Types of examination of the neonate

Birth provides the first opportunity to examine a baby. Information is obtained from this first examination about the current state of the baby, especially its adjustment to extra-uterine existence, the presence of malformations, the effects of antenatal and natal events, the degree of maturity, and to some extent the future prospects of the baby. There are three principal types of examination:

1. An immediate examination at delivery to assess the physiological status of the baby and its preparedness for extra-uterine existence, and to note any gross malformations.
2. A general clinical examination to determine the intactness of the baby and freedom from malformations.
3. An appraisal of the baby's neurodevelopmental status and maturity.

Observation of parent–infant interaction should be made during these examinations.

A technique for the first type of examination, described by Apgar (1953), is now practised in most places. In this method a score of 0, 1 or 2 is given to each of five important physiological parameters (Table 6.1). The lower the total score, the greater the physiological derangement of the baby. The Apgar score should be calculated 1 min after birth and then at later times if indicated.

A score of 7 or more at 1 min indicates a good prognosis for the baby with respect

Table 6.1 The Apgar score

Sign	Score		
	0	*1*	*2*
Heart rate	Absent	Below 100	Over 100
Respiratory effort	Absent	Weak, irregular	Good, crying
Muscle tone	Flaccid	Some flexion of extremities	Well flexed
Reflex irritability (catheter in nose)	No response	Grimace	Cough or sneeze
Colour	Blue, pale	Body pink Extremities blue	Completely pink

to mortality and subsequent neurological abnormality. Low scores at 1 min are associated with a high mortality (8% for scores of 2–3 and 23% for scores of 0–1) and a high risk of neurological abnormality at 1 year in the survivors (3.6% for scores of 0–3). Low scores persisting to the 5th min are even more ominous: scores of 2–3, mortality 30%; 0–1, mortality 49%; and 0–3, neurological abnormality at 1 year 7.4% (Drage and Berendes, 1966).

Methods of clinical examination both general and neurological have been described many times elsewhere (e.g. Dargassies, 1954; Thomas, Chesni and Dargassies, 1960; Paine, 1961; Prechtl and Beintema, 1968; Brazelton, 1973). The main features of such an examination are summarized below.

(a) Measurement of weight and head circumference (the maximum circumference passing through occiput and just above the bridge of the nose). As the head circumference is measured, opportunity is taken to palpate the fontanelles and sutures. Although measurement of length is useful it is not recommended by some because of the difficulty in getting a reliable measurement, which requires at least two people, and the risk of damage to the baby's hips by over-strenuous attempts to obtain full extension of the legs. The expected length, weight and head circumference measurements for pre-term and term babies are shown in Figure 6.1.

(b) Confirmation of the intactness and normal function of the body systems, especially respiration and circulation, including palpation of the peripheral pulses.

(c) Detection of any congenital malformations, searching particularly for those which can be easily overlooked, namely:

(i)   the eyes for cataract;
(ii) the hips for undue laxity;
(iii) the genitalia and anus for malformation;
(iv) the spine for irregularities and dermal sinuses;
(v)   the various minor malformations which when several are present together indicate the likely presence of a major malformation (Smith, 1970).

The existence, intensity and significance of interaction between parents, especially mothers, and their newly born baby have been described by several workers, particularly Klaus and Kennell (1976, 1982). They showed that babies who do not experience bonding in the early neonatal period do not progress as well as those who do.

Interactions occur between parents and baby; these are multi-sensorial and include touch, warmth, odour, eye-to-eye contact, movement and voice; the interactions proceed in both directions, i.e. from parent to baby and baby to parent; there is a sensitive period for a short time after birth when these interactions lead to bonding; and successful bonding is beneficial.

In the examination of the neonate, note should be made of the adequacy of the interactions and steps taken to remove any barriers to bonding.

Examination of the neonate's eyes is often best done during feeding when the eyes may open. It should not be necessary to force the lids apart nor to use mydriatics. Ophthalmoscopic examination is not part of a routine examination of the neonate, but if it is decided to perform such an examination it is usually possible and even easy to do so while the baby is sucking at a bottle.

A light shone into the eye produces a red reflection from the retina, observation of which confirms that the lens is clear. If the baby is held up in the arms it is possible to demonstrate first automatic turning towards light, and second, after two

64

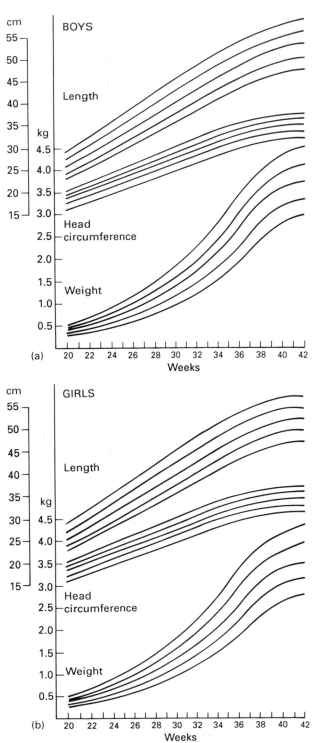

Figure 6.1 Growth record for infants
in relation to gestational age:
(a) boys; (b) girls. Growth parameters:
means +1 and +2 SD (Keen and
Pearse, 1988)

or three rotations, the occurrence of coarse nystagmus, indicating visual function and eye movements.

The hips are examined by Barlow's (1962) modification of the Ortolani test in the following way. The baby lies supine. The examiner stands at the feet, facing the baby. He places each hand on the corresponding shin causing full flexion of the knees and flexion of the hips to a right angle. In this position he can place the middle fingers of each hand firmly over the greater trochanters and the thumbs over the lesser trochanters (Figure 6.2). Each leg is held steady in turn while the opposite leg is abducted. At or just beyond mid-abduction, inward pressure is exerted by the middle finger. If the hip is dislocated the femoral head will be felt to slip over the aectabular lip when this manoeuvre is performed.

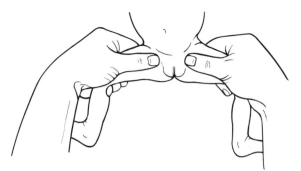

Figure 6.2 Examination of hips for instability and dislocation

Appraisal of the neurodevelopmental status of the neonate is particularly interesting to paediatricians because of the wealth of neurological activity which can be seen, and the clues which it provides to later development. It is an exacting type of examination which enables the paediatrician to estimate the maturity of the baby and to detect discrepancies which might lead to later difficulties and delays in development. Many of the responses observed during the examination are affected by the state of the baby and by external circumstances (e.g. time after feeding, temperature, draughts), and the examination should be done at the most appropriate stage of alertness of the baby. Prechtl and Beintema (1968) described

Table 6.2 Classification of state of neonates (Prechtl and Beintema, 1968)

State of neonate	Criteria considered			
	Eyes	Respiration	Movements	Crying
1	Closed	Regular	None	–
2	Closed	Irregular	No gross movements	–
3	Open	–	No gross movements	–
4	Open	–	Gross movements	No crying
5	Open or closed	–	–	Crying
6	Any state not classifiable as 1–5			

an exceptionally careful technique. Their criteria and classification of the baby's state are shown in Table 6.2.

In a clinical setting it is not always possible to carry out such thorough examinations. Nevertheless paediatricians should have opportunities to do so in their training, so that they become familiar with all that they reveal and are also able to judge the limitations of abbreviated examinations, which they may have to resort to in practice.

The principal features of the examination are as follows:

1. *Alertness of the baby* is determined by noting the general responsiveness, spontaneous movements, respiratory pattern, feeding behaviour, and the strength and promptness of the rooting reflex. This information is used both to judge the state of the baby and as a background against which to evaluate the observations of the rest of the examination. Persistently reduced alertness indicates possible abnormality.
2. *Symmetry of responses* is noted with regard to the range of joint movement, reactions of muscles and pattern of reflexes, having first made sure that the baby is in a symmetrical position at the beginning and throughout the examination. Persisting asymmetry indicates probable abnormality.
3. *Range of movement* is estimated at certain joints, as shown in Table 6.3. Persisting definite variations indicate possible abnormalities. Reduced range of

Table 6.3 Range of movement at certain joints

Movement	Normal response
Rotation of head on shoulders	Chin to acromial tip
Movement of arm across chest (scarf sign)	Fingers to opposite acromial tip
Extension of arm at elbow	180°
Flexion of wrist	150°
Abduction of flexed hips	Approx. 75° each side
Extension of leg at knee when flexed to 90° at hips	Approx. 150°
Dorsiflexion of foot	Approx. 120°

movement is usually due to increased muscle resistance. Increased range of movement may be due to hypotonia or to immaturity. Sometimes variations occur as a result of the position *in utero*. For example, the findings on examination in the first few days of a baby born by breech with extended legs are different from those on a baby born by vertex.

4. *Muscle responsiveness to stretch* is examined with respect to both slow and fast movements. Slow stretch should not produce resistance. If this occurs it is probably abnormal. Rapid repeated stretching of a muscle does produce resistance normally, so that after three or four beats the movement tends to be arrested. This is the basis of the French test for *'passivité'*. Reduced resistance to rapid stretch which permits the hand or leg to continue to swing freely usually indicates immaturity or abnormality.
5. *Neonatal reflexes.* Some of the more easily elicited and useful ones are examined. Abnormality might be indicated by their absence or exaggeration or asymmetry.

Interpretation of the neurodevelopmental examinations

It is unwise to make any interpretation on the basis of finding a single abnormal item. This situation seldom occurs, however, and usually the findings fall into one of three patterns – normal, immature and abnormal.

The criteria for judging neonatal maturity are summarized in Tables 6.4 and 6.5.

Table 6.4 Some criteria of neonatal maturity (Holt, 1963, 1965; Brett, 1965; Farr *et al.*, 1966; Robinson, 1966; Amiel-Tison, 1968; Dubowitz and Goldberg, 1970)

Criteria	Gestational age			
	28 wk	*32 wk*	*36 wk*	*40 wk*
POSTURE				
Arms	Limp, abducted, extended	Extended	Flexed weakly	Flexed strongly
Legs	Limp, abducted, extended	Abducted and flexed	Flexed and less 'frog like'	Flexed strongly
Head	Lateral	Lateral	Maybe control	Control
SPONTANEOUS ACTIVITY				
General	Always	Always	Sometimes	Sometimes
Persists with other activity	Yes	Sometimes	No	No
Individual limbs	Never	No	Sometimes	Yes
FEEDING BEHAVIOUR				
Ease of stimulation	Very difficult	Difficult	Fairly easy	Easy
Response	Feeble	Slow	Fairly brisk	Brisk
Persistence	None	Slight	Fairly good	Good
RANGE OF MOVEMENT				
Head rotation	Well past acromion	Rather less	Rather less	To acromion
Scarf sign	Well past acromion	Rather less	Rather less	To acromion
Hips	Foot to ear	Rather less	Leg vertical	Leg vertical
Knees (popliteal angle)	140–150°	About 110°	About 100°	90° or less
Feet (dorsiflexion)	About 120°	Rather more	Rather more	Onto front of shin
Wrist (flexion)	About 100° (window)	Rather less	Rather less	Acute angle
REFLEXES				
Sucking	Weak	Stronger	Strong	Strong
Rooting	Weak and slow	Stronger	Strong and quick	Strong and quick
Grasp:				
(a) Response	Feeble	Slow	Easier to obtain	Brisk
(b) reinforcement	None	Little or none	Incomplete	Good
Crossed extension:				
(a) flexion	Weak	Present	Present	Present
(b) extension	Absent	Weak	Present	Present
(c) adduction	Absent	Absent	Absent	Present
Moro	Weak	Feeble	Stronger	Strong
Pupillary	Absent	Present	Present	Present
Head turning	Absent	Present	Present	Present
Traction	Absent	Feeble	Present	Present
Glabellar tap	Absent	Present	Present	Present
Neck righting	Absent	Absent	Present	Present

Table 6.5 Some other neonatal criteria scored for maturity (Farr et al., 1966)

Body feature	Grade of maturity				
	0	*1*	*2*	*3*	*4*
Skin texture	Very thin, gelatinous feel	Thin, smooth	Medium thick, smooth	Thickening stiff feel, cracking and peeling	Thick, parchment-like, cracking
Skin colour	Dark red	Uniformly pink	Pale pink, variable	Pale, only extremities pink	–
Skin opacity	Numerous veins seen	Veins seen	A few large vessels clear	A few large vessels indistinct	No vessels seen
Oedema	Obvious	No obvious tibial pitting	None	–	–
Lanugo	None	Abundant	Thinning	Area of baldness	Over half back bald
Skull hardness	Soft	Springy	Some hard, some springy	Hard but displaceable	Hard, not displaceable
Ear form	Flat, shapeless	Some incurving	More incurving	Incurving of all upper pinna	–
Ear firmness	Soft, easily folded,	Soft, easily folded slowly returns	Cartilage palpable, springs back after folding	Firm, definite cartilage	–
Breast size	Nothing	Tissue palpable up to 0.5 cm	0.5–1.0 cm	>1.0 cm	–
Nipple	Barely seen, no areola	Well defined + areola	Well defined + areola raised	–	–
Plantar skin	No creases	Faint creases	Creases indent <1/3 sole	Creases indent >1/3 sole	Definite deep creases
Genitalia	No testes in scrotum; labia maj. widely separated, labia min. large	One testis in scrotum; labia maj. almost cover labia min.	One testis at least well down; labia maj. cover labia min. completely	–	–

Table 6.4 lists various characteristics at four-week intervals between the ages of 28 and 40 weeks. Table 6.5 (Farr *et al.*, 1966) lists other characteristics each of which is given a score of 0–4 according to maturity. The higher the scores for each individual item and for all items together, the greater the maturity of the infant. A total score of 10 or less indicates a gestational age of 32 weeks or less; a score of 21 or over indicates a gestational age of 38 weeks or more; and scores between 11 and 20 indicate gestational ages of 32–38 weeks.

The finding of abnormalities alerts paediatricians to the need for continued observation and, possibly, treatment, and to the risk of persisting disability. Despair is never justified at this stage because even the neonate with the most markedly abnormal examination may make surprisingly good progress. The observations of Dargassies (1971) are interesting in this connection. She followed up 130 babies who had very abnormal findings on neonatal examination and found that at 2 years of age 82 were abnormal, but the other 48 appeared to be normal.

The abbreviated and modified neurodevelopmental examinations which have to be used by most clinicians do not detect all abnormalities, and indeed it is probable that, however detailed and painstaking the examinations, not all abnormalities could be detected in this way. To quote Dargassies again, out of a group of 150 babies with normal neonatal examinations, 2 showed abnormalities at 2 years of age. Nor does the usual clinical examination detect the minor changes which Prechtl and his colleagues (Prechtl, 1965; Prechtl and Beintema, 1968) were able to find with their painstaking technique.

They found variations from normal which fell into three groups – the apathetic, hemi-syndrome and hyperexcitable groups – and in these groups there was a higher incidence of neurological abnormalities at 2–4 years to which subsequent problems such as restlessness, epilepsy and learning disorders were thought to be related.

The neonates in the apathetic group spent long periods in state 3 (see Table 6.2), and showed marked depression of motility, resistance to passive movements, and intensity of reflex responses. The hyperexcitable group of neonates showed a tremor when making gross movements. The tremor was of low frequency (6 beats per second) and high amplitude (3 cm). The neonates also showed increased tendon reflexes and a low threshold of excitability of the Moro reflex. Neonates showing the hemi-syndrome had three or more persisting asymmetries. The frequency and significance of these syndromes according to Prechtl and co-workers are shown in Tables 6.6 and 6.7.

Although it is desirable to identify children with such problems as early as possible in order to begin remedial work, the general feeling at present appears to be that it is seldom possible to translate Prechtl's technique from the research laboratory to the clinical field, and also that harm may result from too early labelling of children.

Table 6.6 Frequency of apathetic, hyperexcitability and hemi-syndromes in neonates

Pre- and perinatal conditions	Number and percentage showing syndrome		
	Apathetic	*Hyperexcitability*	*Hemi*
252 babies with obstetric complications	31 (12.3%)	101 (40.1%)	49 (19.4%)
116 babies with uneventful history	4 (3.4%)	16 (13.8%)	0 (0%)

Table 6.7 Frequency of neurological abnormalities at 2–4 yr in relation to presence of Prechtl syndromes in neonatal period

Neonatal state and numbers of babies	Number and percentage with neurological abnormalities at 2–4 yr
150 with syndromes	110 (73%)
102 without syndromes	14 (14%)

References

Amiel-Tison, C. (1968) Neurological evaluation of the maturity of newborn infants. *Archs Dis. Childh.*, **43**, 89

Apgar, V. (1953) A proposal for a new method of evaluation of the newborn infant. *Curr. Res. Anesth. Analg.*, **32**, 260

Barlow, T. G. (1962) Early diagnosis and treatment of congenital dislocation of the hip. *J. Bone Jt Surg.*, **44B**, 292

Brazelton, T.B. (1973) Neonatal behaviour assessment scale. *Clinics Dev. Med. 50.* London: Heinemann

Brett, E. M. (1965) The estimation of foetal maturity by the neurological examination of the neonate. *Clinics Dev. Med. 19.* London: Heinemann

Dargassies, S. Saint-Anne (1954) Methode d'examen neurologique du nouveau-ne. *Étud. néo-natal,* **3**, 101

Dargassies, S. Saint-Anne (1971) Value of assessing clinical neuropathology at birth. *Proc. R. Soc. Med.,* **64**, 468

Drage, J. S. and Berendes, J. (1966) Apgar scores and outcome of the newborn. *Pediatr. Clin. N.Am.,* **13**, 635

Dubowitz, V. and Goldberg, C. (1970). Clinical assessment of gestational age in the newborn infant. *J. Pediat.,* **77**, 1

Farr, V., Mitchell, R. G., Neligan, G. A. and Parkin, J. M. (1966) The definition of some external characteristics used in the assessment of gestational age in the newborn infant. *Devl. Med. Child Neurol.,* **8**, 507

Holt, K. S. (1963) In *The Development of the Infant and Young Child: Normal and Abnormal,* 2nd edn. (ed. Illingworth, R. S.), p. 251. Edingburgh: Livingstone

Holt, K. S. (1965) Age, growth, and maturity of the neonate. *Clinics Dev. Med. 19.* London: Heinemann

Keen, D. V. and Pearse, R. G. (1988) Weight, length and head circumference curves for boys and girls of between 20 and 42 weeks gestation. *Archs Dis. Childh. (fetal and neonate edn),* **63**, 1170–1172

Klaus, M. H. and Kennell, J. H. (1976) *Maternal-infant Bonding.* St. Louis: C. V. Mosby

Klaus, M. H. and Kennell, J. H. (1982) *Parent-infant Bonding,* 2nd edn. St Louis: C. V. Mosby

Paine, R. S. (1961) Neurological examination of infants and children. *Pediat. Clin. N. Am.,* **7**, 471

Prechtl, H. F. R. (1965) Prognostic value of neurological signs in the newborn infant. *Proc. R. Soc. Med.,* **58**, 3

Prechtl, H. F. R. and Beintema, D. (1968) The neurological examination of the full-term newborn infant. *Clinics Dev. Med. 12.* London: Heinemann

Robinson, R. J. (1966) Assessment of gestational age by neurological examination. *Archs Dis. Childh.,* **41**, 437

Smith, D. W. (1970) *Recognisable Patterns of Human Malformations.* Philadelphia: Saunders

Thomas, A., Chesni, J. and Dargassies, S. Saint-Anne (1960) The neurological examination of the infant. *Little Club Clinics 1.* London: Heinemann

Chapter 7

Development in the first year

Changes in the first year and their significance

The changes occurring in the 12 months after birth are remarkable for their nature and magnitude. Babies grow and emerge from the constraints of reflex control of the early months. Their weight trebles, length doubles and head circumference increases by a third. The developmental changes are highly significant because they establish a firm basis for many later skills and activities, and they prepare the individual for an independent existence.

With respect to motor function, the infant goes from a totally dependent neonate to a 1 year old literally standing on his own feet. Visual and auditory stimuli, which initially produced only reflex responses, are found by the infant to convey much information from which he learns to recognize and identify his surroundings. Objects and people become meaningful and tangible. The striking observation of an 8-month-old infant looking for a dropped cube illustrates the beginning of his sense of permanence of objects and of awareness of continuity in his environment.

Whereas a neonate is at the mercy of his environment and has to depend upon his reflexes for preservation, an infant who has begun to recognize his environment begins to react to it and to control it. Thus, he attempts to use objects appropriately, and begins to interact, communicate and modify his responses to people according to the situation.

The acquisition of each new perceptual skill and the performance of each new action during this busy 12-month period appear to follow a characteristic pattern, with each new task calling forth intense concentration while other activities are for the moment inhibited or ignored. For example, early visual awareness is characterized by prolonged visual fixation with suppression of motor activity and response to sounds; and early tactile exploration is such an intense activity that the infant shows little interest in other stimuli. After these initial stages the infant learns to deal with each particular task with less and less effort and shows increasing ability to switch from the task in hand to other tasks and then return to the original one. Ultimately, a stage is reached when the task requires little effort and can be performed quickly. For example, the visual preoccupation of the initial period is ultimately superseded by a quick visual glance; and turning towards a sound each time it is repeated no longer occurs in this later stage because the infant has analysed and identified the first sound stimulus and further interest is lost. At this stage other new tasks can be given attention and attempts be made to link tasks

Table 7.1 Summary of development in the first year

Age (mth)	Gross motor	Vision and manipulation	Hearing and vocalization	Social
1	Gradual development of head control. Movements coarse and jerky	Begins to fixate on nearby familiar objects. Watches mother's face	Cries when hungry or uncomfortable. Quietens or freezes to sounds	Sleeps and feeds. Evokes much affection and accepts this passively
2	Dominance of primary reflexes on posture and movements	Following with eyes. Visually takes 'hold' of objects		Quiets in response to cooing and rocking. Regards nearby face. Smiles in response
3	When raised from supine to sitting, head lag is less noticeable	Holds objects placed in hands momentarily	Response to sounds varies, e.g. dislikes loud harsh sounds, may excite to familiar sounds	Reacts to familiar pleasant situations, e.g. feeding, bathing
4	In prone position, head and chest raised. Later, support taken on forearms	Visually associated reaching develops	Cry pattern more mature. Vocalizes in response to overtures	Likes handling. Feeding now a social activity
5	Feet to mouth. Plays with toes with hands	Recognizes everyday objects, e.g. cup	Turns to sounds	
6	When held upright takes weight through legs	Mature visual following and convergence. Eyes used together; should be no squint	Wider range of vocalization. Chuckles	Spontaneously responsive and smiling
7	Sits with head steady and back straight	Transfers objects, e.g. cubes, from hand to hand	Beginning to imitate rhythms of sounds	
8	Reciprocates with legs. Protective support reflexes of limbs appearing	Looks for dropped objects	Practises vocalization	Beginning to be aware of strangers and to modify responsiveness
9	Stable in sitting position. Sideways and forward support with arms	Moves cover in order to see object. Index finger use appearing	Babbles, uses voice purposefully. Vocal imitation	Responds to adults; plays imitative games
10	Attempts to move – creep, crawl, squirms, shuffle. Pulls to stand	Visually very alert. Pincer grip for small objects	Mature localization of sounds	Reacts to encouragement and discouragement
11	Plays standing holding on. Cruises around furniture	Glances around, makes quick visual appraisals. Beginning to look at pictures and may point with index finger	Beginning to understand words and single simple commands. Beginning to vocalize recognizable words	Shows affection. Plays pat-a-cake; waves bye-bye
12	May take first steps			

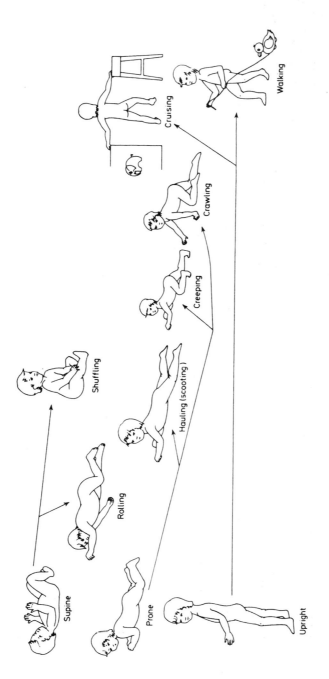

Figure 7.1 Motor development in prone, supine and upright positions

together. Thus, linking of skills appears towards the end of the first year and develops considerably in the following years.

The physical separation of a baby from his mother occurs at birth. The neonate is still dependent, however, and the purpose of development during the first year is to prepare the infant for independence. This is achieved by the acquisition of mobility and the emergence of his individual personality. At 1 year of age the infant is ready for the second major step forward – emancipation from his mother. The succeeding years are spent in building up this independence. Development in the first year is summarized in Table 7.1.

Gross motor development in the first year

Gesell and Amatruda (1947) described the cephalocaudal (head to tail) progression of early gross motor development. The biological value of this observed sequence is obvious. Early stabilization of the head greatly facilitates survival by making feeding easier, and also enables the child to become aware of the world around him through the use of his eyes and ears. The features of early motor development as they occur in the supine, prone and upright postures are summarized in Table 7.2 and Figure 7.1.

Table 7.2 Features of early motor development in supine, prone and upright postures

Posture	Requirements for progress	Advantages	Disadvantages
Supine	Head flexion and stability. Symmetry. Ability to support trunk in upright sitting	Hands free, facilitating early play and hand–eye co-ordination	A static posture for most, apart from those babies who shuffle
Prone	Head extension and stability. Control of symmetrical tonic neck reflex. Symmetry	Leads to early mobility by hauling or crawling	Hands occupied
Upright	Stability of head and trunk against gravity. Balance and fine control of distribution of body weight	Socially acceptable and effective mobility. Hands free	Time taken to acquire anti-gravity postural control

In the supine posture, the neonate's legs and arms are flexed and when the baby is raised to a sitting position the head lags behind. During the first 3 months the head becomes increasingly stable on the shoulders, so that it begins to be raised in anticipation of being pulled to sitting and it becomes possible to put the baby in a supported sitting position (3–4 months). As independent sitting develops the back, which at first is rounded, becomes more erect, and the legs, which at first are widespread giving a broad, stable base, come closer together. The appearance of protective reflexes at 8–9 months provides further stability in sitting. As confidence develops, many children enjoy the sitting position because it leaves their hands free for play and exploration. Sitting is usually a static position and many infants appear happy to sit as unmoving masters of their little play area. A few infants, however, move by shuffling on their bottoms. Robson (1970) claims that there is a familial tendency to bottom-shuffling. Bottom-shufflers acquire independent walking later than other children. From sitting, some infants fall forwards to assume a crawl position and some lean forwards to hold on to a firm object and then contrive to pull themselves to standing.

In the first few months, head stabilization also occurs in the prone posture, but this is achieved by extension of the neck and not with flexion as occurs with head stabilization in the supine posture. Ability to support the chest on, first, the forearms and then on the hands develops next. At this stage the baby in prone posture is much more proficient above the waist than below so far as motor skills are concerned. Some babies even acquire an ability to pull themselves forwards or push themselves backwards with their arms – actions known as *hauling* or *scooting*. Occasionally the discrepancy between upper and lower parts of the body is so marked that an abnormality is suspected, but provided that a neurological disorder is excluded parents can be reassured that locomotor development will occur (Hagberg and Lundberg, 1969).

The prone posture is well adapted to movement. Movement involving both arms and legs and with the trunk on the floor is known in the UK as *creeping*, and it usually occurs before *crawling* in which the trunk is held off the floor and supported by all four limbs. Crawling can be a most effective means of movement, but if the infant wants to use his hands he must stop and fall back to a sitting position. From a crawl position some infants are able to pull themselves to standing.

The upright posture is an anti-gravity posture, so infants have to be held supported in this position in their early months. Initially a stepping reflex can be elicited. This is not true walking because there is no pelvic stability. The reflex is suppressed, and replaced at about 6 months of age by a positive supporting reflex in which the lower limb muscles contract and turn the legs into very good supporting pillars. In this way the infant is helped to acquire a sense of anti-gravity balance, and to learn to maintain an upright posture with less and less muscle effort. Increasing confidence when standing with support or holding on to a firm object enables the infant to make movements of the legs which lead to *cruising* (side-stepping). From this point the infant progresses to independent standing and to taking his first steps. Both cruising and pulling to standing are important actions, for they promote strength and stability of the hip musculature. From standing, an infant can drop to sitting or crawling postures, but, in most instances, once a child is on his feet he wants to be off walking and exploring.

In normal individuals development in the different postures – prone, supine and upright – occurs simultaneously and the child is able to change from one posture to another very easily. Progression to a new ability, it is suggested, occurs as a result of progression from a previous motor activity in the same posture and not necessarily as a result of a previously exhibited motor skill in a different posture. For example, bottom-shuffling develops as a progression from earlier activities in supine and sitting postures, and not because of a previous ability to scoot; nor does shuffling prepare a child for future ability to crawl.

The fact that a motor skill arising in one posture does not necessarily prepare for the development of a motor skill based upon another posture is further supported by a consideration of the muscles involved and the kinaesthetic stimuli arising from the different actions. For example, compare the sitting posture at 9 months with the crawl posture at the same age. In the former, the short hip extensor muscles are relaxed and only contract briefly if they are required for postural support, whereas in the latter they have to be prepared to contract alternately to extend the thigh at the hip whenever crawling is attempted. The muscles are used quite differently, and the kinaesthetic stimuli are different in the two situations. Recognition that early motor development is composed of progress in the supine, prone and upright postures makes it easier to understand (and to accept) the facts that the pattern of motor development may vary from child to child, and that some features of motor development may be omitted altogether even in perfectly normal children. All children do not have to go through all the stages of sitting–crawling–standing in a strict order. Nor does there seem to be any justification for forcing a child to do so because, it is thought, erroneously, that failure to follow a set pattern accounts for some disability at a later age.

Most children follow a fairly similar pattern of early motor development. Those who follow a less common pattern should be examined carefully because there is a greater incidence of motor abnormalities in this group. Nevertheless, some who show deviant motor patterns are perfectly normal and the recognition of this fact can save much parental anxiety and distress. Normal variations of early motor development have been studied by Robson (1984), and he has now described the ages at which children exhibiting these variations acquire the important abilities of standing and walking (Table 7.3).

Gross motor development is directed towards two ends: the attainment of stable positions, especially against gravity as described above, and the achievement of movement. For most children, movement opens up many avenues of development (Table 7.4). Each type of movement has advantages and disadvantages.

Table 7.3 The influence of early motor patterns on ages for sitting, crawling, standing and walking (Robson, 1984)[*]

Motor activity	Early walkers (approx. 85–90% of children)		Late walkers (approx. 10–15% of children)		
	'Just stands and walks'	Crawlers	Rollers	Creepers	Shufflers
Sitting	5–7–11	5–7–9	6–8–10	6–9–12	7–12–15
Crawling	–	6–9–12	11–14–17	12–15–19	–
Shuffling	–	–	–	–	7–12–16
Getting to standing	8–10–13	7–10–13	12–15–20	11–19–24	10–18–26
Walking	8–11–14	11–13–15	14–18–26	15–20–27	12–19–28

[*] The figures refer to ages in months and are given in the order: initial–mean–limit ages

Table 7.4 Advantages of mobility in infancy

Physical	(a) Enhanced physique – circulatory effects, increased muscle strength, etc.
	(b) Practice in development of skills – sensory, motor co-ordination, balance, etc.
Intellectual	(a) Exploration – spatial awareness, promotion of audiovisual development, increased learning opportunities, etc.
	(b) Communication – more effective, wider scope, etc.
Emotional	(a) Internal stimulation and enjoyment
	(b) Interpersonal relationships enhanced and controlled

Rolling
The great limitation of this movement is that it is not possible for the child to look in the direction of movement or at the object he is moving towards all the time, whereas in other forms of movement the child is able to do so. For most children, therefore, rolling is an early transient form of movement which may occur accidentally or be indulged in for pleasure. It might be used occasionally for the purpose of moving to another point or to reach an object. Some disabled children have to use this as their only means of movement, and in these cases its limitations, and therefore their difficulties in making this a functionally useful movement, must be kept in mind.

Scooting, creeping and crawling
All these actions involve the active use of the legs and arms. Consequently, although they can become very effective means of movement, their usefulness is limited by the fact that the hands are not free. It is difficult for a child to carry anything with him as he crawls, and if he wishes to use his hands for exploration, he has to stop and change to another position.

Pulling to standing, cruising and walking
Pulling to standing requires considerable strength, especially in the hip extensors, and difficulty here may provide a useful clinical clue to muscle weakness. The hands are occupied in pulling to standing and cruising. It is not always realized that cruising requires a somewhat unique side-stepping ability which needs good control of the pelvis. Walking, of course, is the one action parents wait for and acclaim with great joy. The prospects opened up by the development of independent walking are considerable. It is a mature and socially accepted means of progression; considerable distances can be explored; the hands are free for manipulation and carrying; progress is visually directed and controlled without difficulty; and it leads to other skills such as running, jumping, hopping, etc.

Sensory development in the first year

Living organisms survive by coming to terms with their environment. They are able to do so by possessing, from an early stage, means of warning to avoid accidents and predators; methods of finding and obtaining food; and ways of learning about their environment. Human beings, like all other organisms, also acquire these biological characteristics.

Infants possess the senses of vision, hearing, touch, smell and taste. Many of the responses of the very young child to sensory stimuli are survival mechanisms, but as the peripheral organs which receive stimuli and the perceptual processes of the brain which analyse and comprehend the sensory input develop, more complex reactions appear and the child is able to build up an increasingly wide range of information about the surrounding world.

Fundamental characteristics of the senses
The eyes respond to waves from the infra-red to the ultra-violet parts of the light spectrum. They are able to receive stimuli from considerable distances, and can distinguish between two points separated by a distance so small that it would subtend at the eye an angle of only 1' (at a distance of 6 m the two points would be separated by 1.74 mm). They can examine near objects and detect fine detail. Eye

movements increase the range of vision. Accommodation and convergence develop to permit frequent, almost instantaneous changes between close and distant viewing. In the older child, colours can be distinguished.

The ears respond to sound waves within the range of 20–20 000 Hz (cycles/s). Their principal role is the detection of speech sounds within the range of 60–8000 Hz. The various speech sounds are produced at different frequencies and intensities. Most vowel sounds have a frequency of below 2000 Hz, and they are produced with energies of 20–30 dB. Consonant sounds are produced over a range of frequencies from 500 to over 8000 Hz. They have less intensity than vowel sounds, and the high-pitched sounds such as 'f' and 'th' are especially weak.

To understand speech a child has to be able to detect sounds of short duration and to recognize differences between sounds in frequency, duration and rhythm. Martin and Martin (1973) studied auditory perception in a group of schoolboys. They found that differences of frequency of 10 Hz and of duration of 200 ms were detected readily, but not so with smaller differences. Sheridan (1958) summarized the situation aptly as follows:

> Every ordinary spoken phrase imposes upon the listening ear the necessity to appreciate a large number of complex sounds which swing rapidly over differences of 8 octaves in pitch and 30 decibels in intensity. For practical purposes one may assume that a quiet voice at 3 feet carries to the listening ear sound intensities varying between peaks at 60 dB and troughs at 30 dB.

In addition, to utilize auditory sensation to the full, children must also learn to listen and to localize the source of sounds.

The sensory organs for *smell* respond to stimuli from varying distances according to their nature, intensity and air currents. Although this sensation is not as well developed in humans as in some other species, it sometimes evokes strong reactions, as when children react to the smell of their food or to a perfume. The sense of smell becomes more important when other distance receptors – vision and hearing – are impaired. For example, the mother of a deaf-blind baby should use the same perfume all the time so that she can be identified easily by her baby.

The senses of *touch* and *taste* are used for nearby and not distant exploration. Tactile sensations consist of touch, pressure, temperature and pain. Sensitivity to tactile stimuli varies in different parts of the body. Areas used for exploration, such as the finger tips, are provided with a greater concentration of nerve receptors than other parts of the body.

The sense of *taste* is fairly crude. It is said to be possible to identify sweet, sour, salt and bitter, but most tastes produce composite pleasant or unpleasant reactions.

The perceptual part of sensation

The peripheral sense organs are useless without the perceptual function of the brain. From the many stimuli he receives, a baby has to learn to identify, distinguish and select those which are most useful to him for self-preservation and learning about the world around himself, and then having selected, he has to learn to suppress irrelevant stimuli. Perceptual development is a demanding task; in the early stages babies tend to be wholly preoccupied with one single sensory channel at a time, to the exclusion of other interests and activities. A good example of preoccupation with one sensory input occurred when I tried to give a demonstration of auditory responses before a rather heavily-jewelled audience. The infants were so visually attracted and occupied that the demonstration was unsuccessful!

The stage of single sensory input concentration passes and then the infant can devote more time to other important learning processes associated with sensory function, such as the simultaneous use of more than one sense for a particular task; rapid switching from one sense to another; and the simultaneous use of two or more senses for different tasks.

Sensory functions equip a child to learn about the world around himself. Impairment of any of these functions impedes this process. Developmental paediatricians are concerned with learning about the complex mechanisms of sensory perceptual development and integration, and with the application of this knowledge to help children in whom these functions are impaired. It is not just a matter of deciding if a child has difficulty seeing or has a hearing loss or not, but of understanding how these losses affect him and what needs to be done to ensure full development despite the losses.

Auditory function

The peripheral auditory sense organs develop early in fetal life, and are probably functional towards the end of pregnancy. There are many stories of fetuses *in utero* responding to external sounds (e.g. Walker, Grimwade and Wood, 1971).

Babies are born into a noisy world. The loudness of some everyday sounds is shown in Table 7.5. Sounds of different intensities arrive at babies' ears from varying distances. Sudden loud noises provoke blinking, grimacing and even crying. Quieter sounds, especially steady notes, appear to be soothing. If everything is kept as quiet as possible, it is not difficult to show that a baby is aware of nearby sounds. Babies show the most consistent responses to sounds when they are made within a conical receptive area extending outwards from the infant's ears. It is difficult for an infant to receive sounds when there is a lot of background noise.

Table 7.5 Intensity of some everyday sounds

Everyday sound	Approximate intensity (dB)
Whisper	15
Average comfortable house	30
Average comfortable office	40
Quiet car	50
Conversation	60
Busy street	70
Cocktail party	75
Loud shout or scream	80
Pneumatic drill	80
Train	90
Engine room	100
Jet engine	110
Thunder	120

Infants become familiar with certain sounds, especially those accompanied by pleasant experiences and those repeated frequently. The mother's voice and certain recurring household noises, such as the clink of crockery, are obvious examples of frequently repeated sounds. Examples of sounds accompanied by other pleasant experiences are the mother's voice followed by gentle caressing and the rattling of a spoon in a cup associated with the pleasures of feeding. Some sounds appear to be more attractive to babies than others. The mother's voice of higher pitch and greater musicality than the father's usually receives more attention from baby. All these examples show the importance of the mother's voice in the early development of an infant's awareness of sounds.

The developing awareness of sounds is linked with turning of the eyes and head towards the side of the sound. This directional response is reflex at first, and is initiated by the reception of auditory stimuli earlier and more intensely on one side than on the other side. Turning of the eyes may be seen occasionally as early as 4 or 5 weeks, even in babies with poor vision, so it must not be taken as an indication of visual ability. As mentioned above, eye and head turning to sound should not be assumed to indicate good vision, and Sheridan (1973) stressed the importance of testing visual fixation and following before testing responses to sounds, in order to reduce misinterpretation of findings. Consistent signs of turning of the head towards sounds appear at about 4 months of age, and visual recognition of the sound-producing object soon follows. Sometimes babies appear to be reluctant to turn towards a sound, but if they are first shown the sound source, e.g. a rattle, they then appear to be more ready to turn towards the sound of that rattle when the test is repeated.

In the six-month period from 4 to 10 months remarkable development occurs in the response of turning towards sounds, which is related to increasing awareness of sounds as distinct entities coming from a source at a definite location. The maturation of auditory localization develops simultaneously with the acquisition of an awareness of the permanence of objects, and the correspondence between these phenomena will be obvious.

The developmental progression in acquiring more precise accuracy in sound localization was described by Murphy (1962). There is a distinct two-phase action in which the baby first turns to the side of the sound and then makes a second movement of the head upwards or downwards towards the sound. Downward localization appears to develop before upward. These two movements gradually merge first into an arc-like movement towards the sound and then a single direct movement which by 10 months localizes the sound to within about 5° (Figure 7.2).

By this time, the ability to hear a sound and to turn directly towards it is no longer a simple reflex action. There has developed the concept of a sound and an ability to inhibit the response. For example, a turning response may not occur if the infant is engrossed visually or tactilely, or if the sound is too familiar or uninteresting.

At this stage the infant is learning to identify and recognize sounds by their intensity, pitch, duration and association with other sounds and events, which, as described earlier, he must become able to do very quickly in order to be able to distinguish all the meaningful sounds of speech. Learning the characteristics of sounds greatly reinforces interest in sounds and promotes the development of auditory attention and listening. The development of auditory alertness and the ability to listen is one of the most important attributes of the infant in the second half of his first year (Fisch, 1971).

Failure to develop auditory interest and listening ability may be due to deafness, or to growing up in an environment which is noisy, or which has little meaningful or interesting auditory stimulation. Such deprivation has a profound effect upon the development of language. In normal circumstances the most frequently heard sounds and also the most interesting ones should come from the human voice.

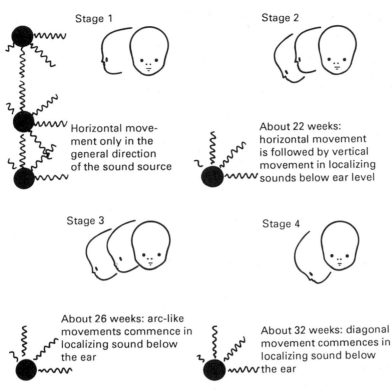

Stage 1

Horizontal move-
ment only in the
general direction
of the sound source

Stage 2

About 22 weeks:
horizontal movement
is followed by vertical
movement in localizing
sounds below ear level

Stage 3

About 26 weeks: arc-like
movements commence in
localizing sound below
the ear

Stage 4

About 32 weeks: diagonal
movement commences in
localizing sound below
the ear

Figure 7.2 Maturation of localization of sounds

Consequently close proximity to the speech source is important at the early stage when auditory discrimination is developing. Children usually listen to their mother's voice on their laps. Once they are mobile and move away from their mother, it is less easy for them to do so. A child playing at the far side of the room will be able to hear his mother's voice, but may not be able to distinguish the various speech sounds at that distance. He then loses interest in verbal communication. Many children are ready, from the point of view of auditory awareness and discrimination, for this distance separation when they achieve independent mobility, but some are not, and in consequence they may suffer a delay in their language development. Parents may not appreciate these issues, and when their child seems to be uninterested in what they are saying they resort to shouting to them (and at them).

Early visual awareness and exploration

The essential visual element of the human eye – the retina – consists of two parts. The major, peripheral part is spread out as a bowl-shaped light-sensitive receptor which is especially responsive to changes of light intensity and movement. The small, centrally situated part – the macula – is specialized for fine discriminative vision.

The peripheral retina is anatomically and functionally well developed at birth. A sudden increase in light intensity or a quick movement near the eyes causes the baby to blink protectively. This reflex mechanism soon becomes extremely sensitive and thereafter persists throughout life. The response may be so sensitive that the slightest movement or shadow in the peripheral visual field of a deaf infant during testing produces a response which may be interpreted erroneously as due to the test sound.

The macula is not as well developed at birth as the surrounding retina, but it soon becomes so. In the early weeks, a baby fixes his gaze upon objects of moderate size situated about 0.3–0.6 m (1–2 ft) away from the eyes and clearly distinct from the background, such as when objects are suspended on a string or placed on the end of a stick. Slight movement aids fixation, and the more interesting the object (e.g. the more patterned), the longer the duration of gaze (Fantz, 1958). The infant's gaze is often fixed upon his mother's face which possesses these characteristics and, in addition, the most valuable asset of responsiveness. Consequently, what may begin as automatic or reflex visual fixation upon a nearby 'object' at about 5 or 6 weeks of age soon becomes the basis of a deeply significant and satisfying interpersonal relationship. The mother responds to the infant's gaze by animation of her face, movement of her eyes and vocalization. The baby responds to this global situation by smiling, and these actions and responses soon become mutually reinforcing.

The *doll's eye phenomenon* is observed in the first week or two of life. When the baby's head is turned to one side, the eyes lag behind. This reaction soon disappears as head and eye positions and movements become associated.

In humans, the visual fields of each eye overlap, so it is essential that the eyes function as a single visual unit. The combined effective field of vision is available to explore the world to the front and sides of the child, but not posteriorly. Early fixation promotes conjugate action of the eyes which is further enhanced as visual following movements develop.

When an object upon which visual fixation has been obtained is moved slowly to one side, the eyes move to maintain visual fixation up to the limit of movement. When fixation is lost, the eyes return to their resting position. Such visual following occurs first in a horizontal plane over a limited range. The range of following increases rapidly with age, and simultaneously there appears the ability to follow in vertical and oblique directions. Variations occur from infant to infant and so rigid criteria cannot be laid down, but any marked delay in fixation and following, and any failure to make progress, must be regarded with suspicion. Fixation and some horizontal following should be demonstrable at 6–8 weeks, and following in all directions should be well established by 6 months.

The early ability to visually fixate and follow is utilized in clinical tests of visual acuity in the early months of life. When an object consisting of contrasting fine black and white lines, or of black circles on a white background, is moved slowly in front of the eyes, nystagmus is induced, provided that visual fixation upon the contrasting lines or shapes has occurred. The lines or circles are made smaller until fixation no longer occurs and nystagmus cannot be produced. This represents the limit of the infant's visual acuity. This subject was reviewed by Catford and Oliver (1973). Using a specially designed portable nystagmus drum, they estimated that visual acuity in the young child was comparable to 6/18 at 5 months, 6/9 at 18 months, and 6/6 at 3 years.

The value of the abilities to fixate and to follow is greatly enhanced as stability of head posture is obtained. The visual field which the infant can explore is increased by controlled movement of the head and change of bodily position. Even so, the range of the infant's visual interest seems to be limited to a few feet in the early months. If visual fixation is obtained upon an object or person which is then moved further away, the fixation will be lost after the first few feet. This appears to be a cognitive limitation rather than a visual one. The range of visual awareness expands more quickly than the range of auditory awareness.

One of the features of visual development at this early stage is the long steady periods of fixation which are observed. This is presumably a process by which the infant learns to visually identify familiar objects.

The development of visual recognition can be seen quite clearly when the infant gets excited upon seeing his bottle or his mother. The process is stimulated by the linking of visual and tactile sensations. Many of the early tactile sensations occur by chance, as when a sweeping arm knocks the object under observation. If the infant is looking at the object as he knocks it, the possibility of a visual–tactile link developing is present. Opportunities for this to occur at about 2–3 months of age are created by the asymmetrical tonic neck response which ensures that the arm on the side to which the child is looking is extended. From this simple beginning develops the following sequence:

awareness of tactile contact – repetition of action, first accidentally then purposefully – visual control of movements – visual direction of active reaching – correlation of tactile impressions of objects with visual impressions of same object – development of ability to move object into visual field of interest.

Thus the infant rapidly acquires the ability to see–touch–take hold of–and bring towards himself objects within his immediate vicinity. Objects he can see are now in two groups: those he can touch and those which he cannot touch. He is beginning to acquire an awareness of distance and of spatial relationships.

The visual and tactile exploration which has gone on in the early months helps the infant to achieve an awareness of the permanence of objects in the second half of the first year. This increasing awareness further intensifies his visual searching and many infants are extremely visually alert at this stage. Variations occur, but those who are most alert appear to be searching with their eyes all the time. They will look for every new object in their surroundings and will examine it visually with great preoccupation, often inhibiting responses to other stimuli (e.g. auditory) during this time. They enjoy playing games of looking for hidden objects.

The desire to visually explore stimulates mobility. The development of mobility, however this may be achieved (by rolling, shuffling, crawling, etc.) enhances visual exploration and experiences. By this stage the infant's visuoperceptual world has expanded considerably.

Fine motor development in the first year

Initially the hands are closed most of the time and the grasp reflex controls the responses to anything placed in the palm. The strength of the grasp reflex wanes and the asymmetrical tonic neck reflex (ATNR) develops. The later reflex causes extension of the arm on the side to which the head is turned and leads sooner or later to a chance contact with nearby objects. Normally, the child will be looking at the object, so that there is the opportunity to link visual and tactile sensations. The early arm movements become more purposeful. Decline of the grasp reflex allows the object to be touched and held. The ATNR fades and in doing so allows the arms to come towards the mid-line. Any object which has been taken hold of is now brought towards the face where mouthing, tasting, smelling and close visual inspection enable the child to learn about the object. The central activity of the hands at 5–6 months is quite different from the peripheral manipulative attempts a month or two earlier.

Another result of the movement of the hands towards the body at 5–6 months is that the two hands may come together and feel and manipulate each other. If either hand is holding anything it may pass it to the other hand, and so begins the process of transfer from hand to hand. When both hands are holding something, the objects will be regarded visually and may be knocked together.

At this stage (i.e. around 6 months), objects are held in the palm of the hand. There then develops increasing use of the fingers and of the thumbs which begin to work in opposition to the fingers. Grasp of objects moves from the palms of the hands to the more precise thumb and fingers. The developments at this time can be studied with a few 25 mm (1 in) wooden cubes (Figure 7.3).

(a) The infant's grasp of a cube demonstrates the level of neuromuscular maturation, the disappearance of the grasp reflex, and the development of the

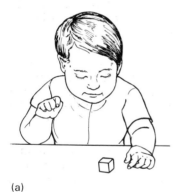
(a)

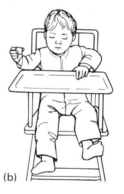
(b)

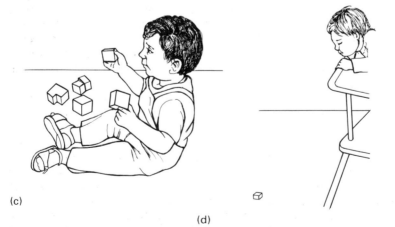
(c)

(d)

Figure 7.3 Manipulation of cubes: (a) tentative approach to one cube; (b) secure thumb–finger grasp of cube in one hand; (c) grasps a cube in either hand and wonders how to use them; (d) looks for dropped cube

control of thumb abduction and opposition. It is difficult to place a cube in a baby's hand in the first few weeks because the effort usually intensifies the grasp reflex and causes the fist to clench even more. A cube can be placed in the hand easily at about 2 months of age. It is retained by a palmar grasp in which the ulnar side of the hand usually takes the larger share. This grasp gradually becomes more certain and by 6–7 months the radial side of the hand plays the predominant role. As the thumb increases in size and can be brought into opposition with the fingers, the grasp upon the cube moves from the palm to between the thumb and fingers.

(b) The strategies involved in taking up one or two cubes reveals much about an infant's perceptual awareness. When it is said that an infant at the age of 5 months shows voluntary grasp, it means that he is visually aware of the cube on the table in front of him and that he can direct his arm and hand into the appropriate position and take hold of it. He does this consistently and without delay by 6 months of age. When there is a second cube on the table, the infant may appear to be unaware of it, or he may be aware of it but do nothing about it, or he may drop the first cube and take up the second with the same hand, or he may transfer the first cube to the opposite hand and then take up the second with the hand which had held the first one, or he may attempt to take up the second cube in the same hand as the first, or he may take up the second cube in his other hand. The possible actions are listed in the order in which they usually occur from 4 to 8 months, but individual babies sometimes show variations in the strategies which they employ.

(c) Study of an infant's reactions to cubes in either hand reveals more areas of developing perceptual awareness. Six months is usually accepted as the age at which most babies demonstrate their ability to transfer an object from one hand to the other. As this ability progresses, infants will take cubes in each hand and then bring them together and compare them. This action may be seen at the age of 8 months, but many more months are required for infants to obtain all the information which is possible from such comparison.

(d) Accidental release occurs early; voluntary release much later. It requires only relaxation of the flexor muscles of the fingers for gravity to cause a cube to fall from the hand. At first the infant takes no further notice of a cube which drops from his hand. Once it has gone it has ceased to exist. At about 8 months of age, a change is observed. The infant begins to search for dropped objects, showing the dawning awareness of their continued existence. Piaget described this important stage as a sense of the permanence of objects. Voluntary release of a cube does not occur until the infant has an awareness of the object he is releasing and can voluntarily relax the flexor muscles. Consequently voluntary release of a cube is not seen until near the end of the first year.

Infants play at giving a cube before they are actually able to do so. An infant with a cube in his hand will push it into the examiner's hand as if giving the cube, but will then withdraw his hand still grasping the cube. As the ability to release develops, the actions of giving, releasing and then withdrawing the hand are crude and exaggerated, but with practice more gentle release becomes possible. Once release is well established, *casting* begins to appear. This consists of the deliberate dropping, pushing and even throwing of objects from the cot, pram or high-chair. It seems as if the infant wants to practise his new motor skill of release and to increase his awareness of space and the permanence of objects. Casting may seem to be an irritating habit, but its developmental value is considerable and is even more important if the mother realizes its value and incorporates casting into play.

(e) Introduction of a cup enables one to explore the child's ability to put cubes into and take them out of the cup, and his ability to detect a cube hidden by a cup. These actions explore developmental levels around 9 and 10 months of age. If an infant aged about 9 months is shown a cube which is then covered by an inverted cup, he will usually attempt to find the cube, revealing his awareness of its presence. Infants aged 10 months will usually take a cube out of a cup, and they may even put one in, but they keep hold of it and do not usually release it until they are a few months older.

Communication in the first year

Babies are not just small dependent individuals who have to be fed and changed and left to sleep. They play an active part in their own early development (Shaffer and Dunn, 1980).

Immediately after birth, close physical contact promotes mother–infant bonding and thereafter both mother and baby promote interaction. Mothers assume responsiveness in babies and act appropriately – hold them closely, look intently at them there, touch them, smile, make noises, rock them. Babies' actions call for notice – they move their heads, arms and eyes, coo and gurgle, change facial expressions and smile. These actions promote responses from even the quietest of mothers. Mothers reinforce and continue their own actions when they get responses from their babies. In these ways, active interaction between the two develops.

Observation studies of 38 everyday activities of 1-month-old babies showed that the mothers vocalized 249 times and the babies responded on 50 of these occasions; and the babies vocalized 136 times and elicited responses from the mothers on 99 occasions. Facial expressions and vocalizations (Condon and Sander, 1974) are especially good stimuli for interaction in the early months.

Whereas the early responses appear to be spontaneous and easily initiated and reinforced, a greater range of control appears in later months. As the infant becomes more aware of his actions, he begins to exercise more control over them. From about 9 months babies become more selective in their responses and interactions.

Ability to vocalize is present at birth, and it is the only means of voice expression in the early months of life. Verbalization develops later and then becomes the principal means of voiced expression, but vocalization is not lost and it remains effective throughout life. For example, it is used as a means of attracting attention by shouting; expressing emotion by roaring with anger or sighing with pleasure; and communicating by cooing to soothe.

Crying

Crying is one form of vocalization. The cry of a newborn infant is quite distinctive, and mothers claim to be able to recognize the cry of their own baby. A trained observer with a keen ear will recognize variations in the cries of normal babies which express different emotions, and also abnormal cries. Wasz-Hockert et al. (1968) studied these differences in infants' cries spectrographically and were able to show that crying is purposive. They distinguished the normal birth cry and the cries of the babies in pain, and when feeling hungry and contented.

The cry pattern changes markedly during the first 2 years of life. The changes appear to follow a definite pattern and presumably occur as a result of alterations in the size and configuration of the oral structures, neuromuscular characteristics and posture of the infant. Karelitz, Karelitz and Rosenfeld (1960) drew attention to these developmental changes.

The first cry is probably the result of the anoxic stimulus following severing of the umbilical cord. In the early days the cry is of very short duration. It seems staccato. If produced by a stimulus such as pinching, the cry rises in crescendo with the stimulus, but then fades, so the stimulus has to be repeated. In consequence, the cry seems very repetitive.

As development proceeds, the duration of each cry lengthens, thereby slowing the tempo and reducing the sense of urgency imparted by the early cry. The rhythmic pattern persists, but is less noticeable because there are more syllables and the pitch is more variable. The inflections seem to be more plaintive and meaningful.

By 2–3 months, cooing and gurgling sounds are heard. These consist of simple sounds at first, but as more sounds are added babbling begins to appear. An expressive 'ah-ha' is added to the cry in the later months.

Appreciation of the cry characteristics at different ages enables one to recognize abnormality and immaturity. Such skill is an invaluable asset to every clinician concerned with babies and infants.

Non-crying vocalizations

The early non-crying vocalizations are variously described as *cooing* and *gurgling*. They are pleasant musical sounds made with the mouth open. The repertoire is increased later by sounds made with the lips at the front of the mouth, often called *buzzing*. It is said that all babies throughout the world produce the same range of these sounds in their early vocalizations, although later they will learn to speak very different languages.

The earliest sounds appear to be produced spontaneously, often to the apparent surprise and pleasure of the child. Within a few months, however, a repetitive element appears in the vocalizations with some of the sounds being made at the front of the mouth (e.g. m, b). This is called *babbling*. Congenitally deaf infants seem to vocalize normally at first but it does not persist, and failure of babbling to appear or to continue is one of the early features which alerts parents and paediatricians to the possibility of deafness.

By the 5th and 6th months vocalizations are more complex with two-syllable repetitions such as 'mama' and 'dada'. These vocalizations attract attention and are used frequently and effectively to this end.

By 8–9 months vocalizations are more tuneful, often imitative, and used with facial expressions and gestures to communicate wishes. No longer are they simple interactive responses.

A great advance occurs in the second half of the first year, when the infant begins to imitate sounds. To be able to do this, he must have been exposed to a number of sounds and been able to hear them; to have selected particular ones – perhaps those which were most distinctive or most frequently heard – and to have modified his own vocalizations to match those he had heard. At this stage, interesting little vocal games can be played with infants.

Babies use their crying and non-crying vocalizations as expressions of their present state, crying when wet and uncomfortable or hungry, and gurgling when happy and playful. Perceptive mothers come to recognize the meaning of certain vocalizations. For example, a certain pattern of grunts may mean that the nappy is about to be filled. Some use their vocalizations as a means of communication, especially to get attention. The greater the astuteness of the child, the greater the use he can make of vocalizations. If verbalization does not develop, then much use may be made of vocalizations in communication. Any child who has to rely upon vocalizations should not be condemned as severely retarded, infantile or animal-like until careful study has been made of all aspects of his development.

Vocal play occurs towards the end of the first year, and with some children their first recognizable words appear. *Echolalia* – repetition of sounds – may also develop.

Cognitive development in the first year

By the end of their first year infants can recognize people, objects and situations. Familiar people such as parents and siblings are recognized readily and often by just one or two clues, such as their voice, and unfamiliar people are distinguished without difficulty. Familiar objects excite interest. For example, the sight of a feeding bottle arouses anticipation for feeding and a small hairbrush may be taken and moved to the head in simulation of hair brushing.

Infants recognize when preparations are being made for feeding or going out for a walk. Changes of voice are important guides for them to know whether or not to proceed with their activities. To a cautionary 'no', they will pause and usually then desist in whatever they were doing.

They possess early concepts of space and time. When they see an object, they know whether or not they can reach out for it or have to move nearer to it by, say, crawling. They recognize a certain permanence to their world and that objects are not gone for ever if they slip out of their hands or go beyond their vision.

Emotional development in the first year

The dominance of internal sensations such as hunger and satiation over an infant's feelings in the early months declines and is replaced by responses to external situations.

Spontaneous pleasure is generated by adult overtures. Apprehension can be felt as unfamiliar events and individuals come to be recognized.

Feelings appear to be simple and to relate to the particular moment. Change of mood occurs readily. They recognize discouragement and respond to encouragement. They especially enjoy simple adult-initiated games.

References

Catford, G. V. and Oliver, A. (1973) Development of visual acuity. *Archs. Dis. Childh.*, **48**, 47

Condon, W. S. and Sander, L. W. (1974) Neonate movement is synchronized with adult speech. *Science*, **183**, 99–101

Fantz, R. L. (1958) Pattern vision in young infants. *Psychol. Rec.*, **8**, 43

Fisch, L. (1971) The probability of response to test sounds in young children. *Sound*, **5**, 7

Gesell, A. and Amatruda, C. S. (1947) *Developmental Diagnosis*, 2nd edn. New York: Harper and Row

Hagberg, B. and Lundberg, A. (1969) Dissociated motor development simulating cerebral palsy. *Neuropediat.*, **1**, 187

Karelitz, S., Karelitz, R. and Rosenfeld, L. (1960) Infant vocalisations and their significance. In *Mental Retardation* (eds. Bowman, P. and Mautner, H.). New York: Grune and Stratton

Martin, J. A. M. and Martin, D. (1973) Auditory perception. *Br. Med. J.*, i, 459

Murphy, K. P. (1962) Ascertainment of deafness in children. *Panorama,* Dec. 3. Reading: Linco Acoustics Ltd

Robson, P. (1970) Shuffling, hitching, scooting or sliding. Some observations in 30 otherwise normal children. *Devl. Med. Child Neurol.,* **12,** 608

Robson, P. (1984) Pre-walking locomotor movements and their use in predicting standing and walking. *Child Care Hlth Dev.,* **10,** 317

Shaffer, D. and Dunn, J. (1980) *The First Year of Life.* Chichester: John Wiley

Sheridan, M. D. (1958) *Manual for the Stycar Hearing Test.* Windsor: NFER

Sheridan, M. D. (1973) *Children's Developmental Progress.* Windsor: NFER

Walker, D., Grimwade, J. and Wood, C. (1971) Foetal response to sound. *Am. J. Obstet. Gynec.,* **109,** 91

Wasz-Hockert, O., Lind, J., Vuorenkoski, V., Partanen, T. and Valanne, E. (1968) The infant cry. *Clinics Dev. Med. 29.* London: Heinemann

Chapter 8

Developmental characteristics and examination at certain ages in the first year

Review of development in the first year

6 weeks old

At 6 weeks of age a baby is still a 'babe in arms', and when carried requires adequate support for the head. The general flexed posture still predominates, and limb movements are still gross and purposeless. The fists may be open from time to time. From his usual comfortable, well-wrapped position the 6-week-old explores the world around him with his eyes. His most characteristic response is a steady fixation of gaze upon his mother's face and a spontaneous smile in response to her overtures. He responds to sounds according to their intensity by either quieting or stilling or by a startle response.

When he is laid prone the pelvis may still be high, but the legs are now extended backwards. The head may be raised momentarily (Figure 8.1).

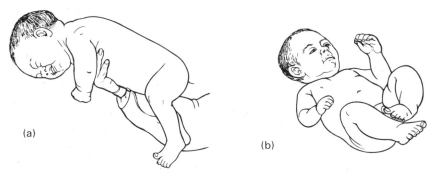

Figure 8.1 Six weeks old: (a) ventral suspension; (b) posture in supine position

When supine, the limbs, especially the arms, may assume an asymmetrical tonic neck reflex posture, with the arm on the face side being extended and the other arm flexed. Head lag is present when he is raised to sitting from supine, but is much less marked than in the earlier neonatal period.

In a supported sitting position the back is smoothly rounded and the head raised momentarily.

When held in ventral suspension the arms and legs are flexed and do not hang down limply, as they did a few weeks earlier, and the head is raised to the same plane as the trunk. When held upright, no appreciable degree of weight-bearing occurs. It is now less easy to elicit a stepping reflex.

Some vocalization may be heard during observation and examination, consisting of some rather guttural grunts of contentment or lusty cries of distress or hunger.

Examination at 6 weeks consists of:

Enquiry about parental concerns, feeding, sleeping, bowel actions and micturition (good stream in boys).

Observation of carrying and handling by mother, responsiveness of baby, amount of head support needed, opening of hands. Call (1974) describes, as signs of early learned behaviour: infant's attentiveness visually to mother's smile and auditorily to her voice, anticipatory behaviour at feeding, response to soothing and differentiation of cry related to types of discomfort. He also points out that valuable information can be obtained from the mother's method of holding – lack of support, dependent holding and lack of visual attention indicate maternal depression; stiffness and clutching indicate maternal anxiety.

Measurement of weight and head circumference.

Examination for congenital defects, especially eyes (inspection), heart (ausculta-tion), genitalia (inspection) and hips (manipulation); of posture in prone, supine, pull to sitting, supported sitting, ventral suspension and upright, noting possible abnormal features such as asymmetry, hypotonia and hypertonia, excessive change of tone with change of posture, strongly persisting primary reflexes; of visual fixation and response when gazing at mother's face.

3 months old

Although still very much a baby, considerable control over posture and muscle activity has been acquired in the intervening weeks. Head control is usually good and the mother gives support at the shoulders, rather than behind the head, when lifting the baby. Visual and auditory interests have increased and the eyes move around to look at nearby objects even if the head is not turned.

When supine, the flexed posture is less marked and the limb movements are smoother and more controlled than previously. The hands are loosely open most of the time. Most babies at this age will anticipate being lifted to sitting either by a pleasurable social response, or by tensing the neck muscles and raising the head, or in both these ways. As the baby is raised to sitting, the head should be firm on the shoulders most of the time, with little head lag, if any at all. When held sitting, the back is straight and the head is bobbingly erect (Figure 8.2).

When prone, the pelvis is quite flat and the head and chest are raised for short periods as weight is taken usually on the forearms.

In ventral suspension, limb flexion is now only slight. The head is raised to look forwards.

Visual alertness is considerable. The baby may stare fixedly at nearby objects as if he were 'taking hold of them with his eyes'. He turns his eyes and head to follow moving objects. He also shows awareness of and interest in sounds, and his own vocalizations are becoming interesting coos and gurgles. He begins to recognize familiar people and situations and reacts pleasurably at the sight of his mother, bottle or bath.

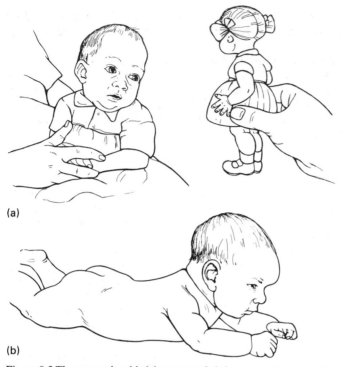

(a)

(b)

Figure 8.2 Three months old: (a) supported sitting – visual interest; (b) posture prone

Examination at 3 months consists of:
Enquiry about parental concerns.

Observation of carrying and handling by the mother. Alertness and vocalizations of the baby.

Measurements of weight and head circumference.

Examination of genitalia (inspection), hips (manipulation) and cardiovascular system (auscultation of heart and palpation of peripheral pulses); of posture in prone, supine, pull to sitting, supported sitting, ventral suspension and upright, noting adequacy of head stability, symmetry of postures and decline of primary reflexes; of visual fixation and following using a bright coloured visual stimulus, e.g. a 50 mm (2 in) diameter ball on string, passed slowly and horizontally about 0.3–0.45 m (12–18 in) in front of the eyes.

The measurement of visual acuity is not part of a routine clinical examination in the first year, although possible methods are the subject of active research (Atkinson and Braddick, 1979; Dobson, 1986). Attention is given to excluding the presence of cataract, gross visual defect and movement disorders. In some cases, however, exploration of visual acuity may be desired.

Two techniques exist for the examination of visual acuity in the early months – the production of optokinetic nystagmus and demonstration of preferential looking.

Alternating vertical black and white lines are moved slowly in front of the baby. He visually fixates upon the stripes and because of the movement nystagmus is produced. The test is repeated with increasingly narrow stripes until nystagmus no longer occurs, indicating that the baby cannot now distinguish the individual stripes. This phenomenon is the basis of the Catford drum test (Catford and Oliver, 1973).

From their early days babies will look longer at a complex pattern than a plain one. By using test cards which differ in pattern by decreasing degrees, it is possible to find a point at which preferential looking occurs no longer, indicating that the baby does not now detect a difference between the test cards. The phenomenon of preferential looking is now used in an acuity card assessment of vision in infancy (Teller *et al.*, 1986; Mohn *et al.*, 1988).

6 months old

By 6 months of age considerable muscle control has been acquired and an infant of this age is able to take up and maintain several different postures. He has acquired some awareness of and familiarity with his immediate environment and is preparing for the development of mobility.

He is seen no longer as a babe in arms, but as a definite individual sitting up in his cot or high-chair, or on his mother's lap. He enjoys the supported sitting and standing postures where he can use his hands, and strives to get out of supine and prone positions.

When supine, he raises his head from the pillow, and with relatively little assistance raises to sitting and sits with a straight back and steady head (Figure 8.3). He may sit alone for a brief moment, and can be sat in a high-chair.

When prone, he raises himself on his extended arms and may show various manoeuvres to move from this position such as *swimming* (with back arched and arms and legs raised), *pivoting* (rotating around on abdomen) and *scooting* (dragging himself forward with his hands).

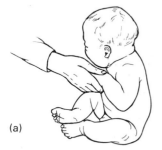

(a)

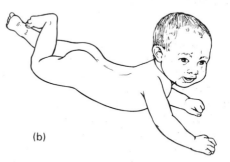

(b)

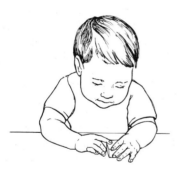

(c)

Figure 8.3 Six months old: (a) supported sitting; (b) prone; (c) manipulation

When he is held upright his legs extend and adduct slightly (parachute reaction); then as the feet contact a firm surface he contracts his leg muscles, turning his legs into strong supporting pillars as he supports most of his body weight. He enjoys this, and bouncing up and down in this position is often a great delight especially at bath time.

He holds his arms out to be lifted up. He reaches out spontaneously and accurately with either hand, taking objects with a palmar grasp and bringing them to the mid-line, and he is beginning to transfer them from hand to hand.

Conjugate movement of the eyes and binocular fixation are now established, so squint is not normally seen after this age. Visually he is busy identifying objects and learning to distinguish them from the immediate environment.

He is interested in sounds, appears able to distinguish familiar from strange noises, and turns towards sounds. His own vocalizations show a wide range of sounds and a tuneful sequence effect called babbling. He is just beginning to show a little coyness with strangers.

Examination at 6 months consists of:

Enquiry about parental concerns, response to sounds, presence of factors producing risk of hearing impairment (Table 8.1), appearance of chewing movements, and progress.

Table 8.1 Babies at risk of hearing impairment

Family history of childhood deafness or malformations of ears, hips or palate

Maternal rubella in pregnancy

Infants with malformations of ears, hips or palate:
    birth weight under 1.5 kg; high bilirubin level in first week (>20 mg/100 mg);
    previous meningitis; recurrent ear infections;
    failed neonatal auditory response cradle;
    and abnormal auroscopic examination

Parents with concerns about child's hearing (Hitchings and Haggard, 1983)

Observation of head control, use of hands, alertness, response to sounds, and vocalizations.

Measurement of weight and head circumference; possibly also length and blood pressure.

Examination (a) of hips, heart and peripheral pulses, motor behaviour in prone, supine, raise to sitting, sitting and upright positions, noting as satisfactory features absence of primary reflexes, good head control, symmetry and presence of positive supportive reflex.

(b) Of manipulation – when he is sitting comfortably supported, offer cube and note reaching and grasp. Check each hand. Note centralization of cube with mouthing and bringing to other hand for transfer.

(c) Of vision – hold visual stimulus (50 mm [2 in] ball on string) 0.45 m (18 in) in front of his eyes and note fixation; move stimulus horizontally and vertically and note range of following and absence of squint and nystagmus; move stimulus towards face and note convergence. Place discreetly on table top in front of baby (a piece of green baize can be placed on table) a small object such as a Smartie or a pellet of rolled-up paper and observe visual fixation and reaching.

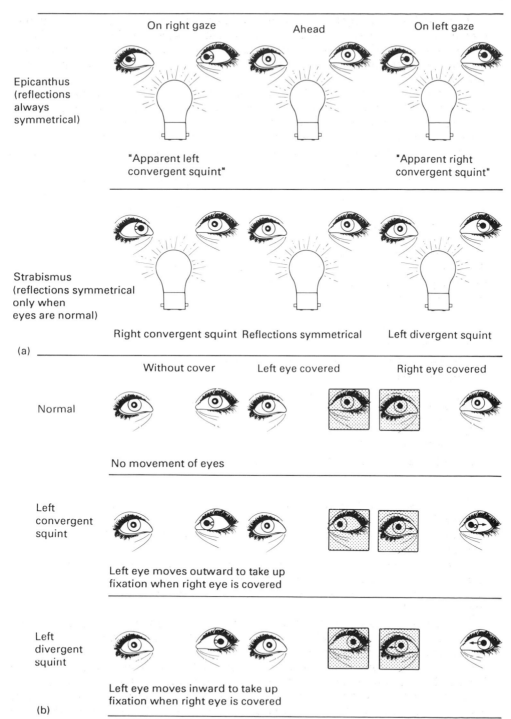

Figure 8.4 Tests for latent strabismus: (a) corneal reflections; (b) cover test (After a poster distributed by Ayerst International, by permission)

Hold a light (e.g. small torch) in front of his face. There should be symmetrical reflections in each cornea. Asymmetry indicates strabismus. The presence of epicanthic folds can give an impression of strabismus and this light test can show the true situation (Figure 8.4a).

The *cover test* (Figure 8.4b) can be performed at this age. The baby's attention is obtained with a visual lure; a hand or card is placed quickly in front of one eye. Note any change of fixation made by the unoccluded eye. The occlusion is now removed – note any change in fixation of the occluded eye. Repeat the test, occluding the other eye. The test reveals inadequate fixation and latent strabismus.

From 6 months onwards the mounted balls test can be used (Sheridan, 1973). The examiner sits behind a black screen in which there is a small slit through which he can observe the baby (Figure 8.5). The baby sits on the mother's knee 3 m (10 ft)

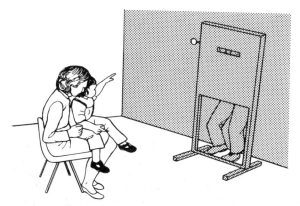

Figure 8.5 Mounted balls test of vision

from the screen or nearer if it is not possible to maintain rapport at the full distance. Balls of different sizes from 3 mm (⅛ in) to 63 mm (2½ in) mounted on thin rods are raised from the screen. If the baby can see the ball, the examiner will note the movement of his eyes as he looks at it. The test will reveal moderate to severe impairment of acuity. Each eye can be tested separately and the mounted balls can be used to test the field of vision.

The balls can be used separately and rolled across the floor to note if the child sees and follows them. Although it was hoped that this procedure could be used as a vision screening test in infancy, it has proved to be unreliable.

(d) Of hearing – by noting the infant's response to sounds which normally consists of turning towards the source of the sound. The theoretical basis of *distraction hearing tests* is misleadingly simple because in practice great care is required to obtain reliable results (Table 8.2).

The room used for the tests must be quiet and free from echo and visual and auditory distractions, but it need not be completely sound free (in fact such a room is difficult to construct, is expensive, and is difficult to work in for long). Reflecting surfaces, shadows and draughts, which might cause distraction and give false-positive responses, should be avoided.

The examiner must be able to move about freely and quietly, hence there must be sufficient space, there must be a carpet on hard floors, and rustling clothes and rattling ornaments must be abandoned. It is necessary to be able to make sounds up

Table 8.2 Factors leading to fallacious results in hearing tests

Hearing normal but deafness suspected because of lack of response

Tiredness or boredom of infant or examiner
Uninteresting or unfamiliar sounds
Use of same sound repeatedly
Making sounds in wrong position
Infant too preoccupied visually or tactilely
Examiner insensitive to minimal and delayed responses

Deafness present but missed because response observed

Infant visually alert and detects movements of examiner or his shadow
Examiner careless and makes movements in infant's visual field or touches infant's hair
Infant responds to draughts or vibrations
Examiner interprets chance movement as response
Assistant gives clues by facial expression

to 1 m (3 ft) or more lateral to either ear, so the room should be at least 3–4 m (10–13 ft) in length.

The infant must be comfortable, sitting usually on mother's lap, and neither too sleepy nor too fretful (Figure 8.6). His attention is attracted by an assistant about 1 m in front of him, who must keep the stimulation at just the right level for the test and avoid excessive visual stimulation or tactile preoccupation with playthings, both of which could lead to false-negative responses in the test. Also, he should not give any signs which might be used as clues by the baby.

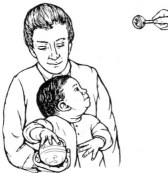

Figure 8.6 Free field distraction hearing test

The sounds are made lateral to and on a level with each ear, at varying distances. Sounds are made on one side or the other in a random fashion to maintain interest and to discourage automatic turning from side to side.

The tests are carried out using a variety of general sounds (e.g. scrape of spoon on cup, rattle, tap on wood, rustle of tissue paper, bell, voiced 's' or 'ff', or pure tones). In actually carrying out the test, the sounds should not be too loud; for example, the spoon should be gently scraped along the inside of the cup (some examiners tap the cup sharply with the spoon, but this is far too loud). It is possible to obtain a rattle which cannot produce sounds of more than 40 dB intensity. During the examination it is useful to have a sound-level meter near the child's ear in order to show the intensity of the sounds being received.

Many sounds used in screening tests cover a wide range of frequencies, so it is quite easy to miss a hearing loss affecting only certain frequencies. Consequently tests with pure tones and some high-frequency voiced sounds should always be included. Several hand-held audiometers are now available and suitable for this purpose.

Adequate time must be allowed between test sounds to permit the infant to respond, and to avoid confusing him. Repetition of the same sound should be avoided because he may become bored and stop responding.

A record is made of the promptness and type of the infant's responses; the maturity of localization; his vocalizations; and of any other features associated with this test.

The factors leading to fallacious results are listed in Table 8.2.

Infants at risk of hearing impairment who have a distraction test of hearing should be declared free of impairment only if the test was carried out with scrupulous care and the responses were unequivocal. Doubtful cases should be re-examined and followed up.

9 months old (Figure 8.7)

One of the most distinctive changes which occur about this age is social responsiveness. Before 9 months, infants are happy to sit contentedly on the floor for periods of 10 min or more and give a spontaneous benign response to all who approach. After 9 months, they show awareness of strangers and their responses are controlled and reserved for those who are familiar to them. The appearance of a stranger with an unusual voice or pair of spectacles can easily precipitate a bout of crying. This is just one aspect of a rapidly blossoming social awareness and responsiveness. A 9 month old enjoys personal attention which he will seek by attracting attention using vocalization or pulling clothes, and will reinforce it by participating in games of imitation, such as hand-clapping, peekaboo and vocal play. He tries to help when being fed. He is aware of the emotional content of speech, especially pleasurable approving sounds and regulatory 'no's'.

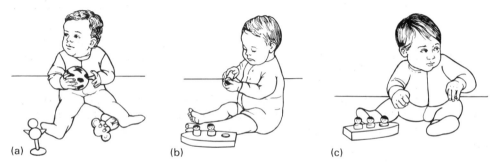

(a)   (b)   (c)

Figure 8.7 Nine months old, sitting: (a) visual interest and ball holding; (b) manipulative play; (c) awareness of strangers

The 9-month-old infant is now more aware of the world around him because he has a concept of the permanence of objects and will look for toys which drop from his hands or from the tray of his high-chair, and he will resist attempts to take a toy away from him. Manipulation is now much more skilful. His fingers are active. The index finger is used to prod and poke; he picks up small objects (e.g. string, Smarties) in a pincer grip between thumb and index finger. He uses his increased manipulative skill to satisfy his exploratory interests in searching for objects inside other containers. He is very stable in independent sitting and may even attempt to shuffle around in this position. He readily changes from sitting to prone, from where he moves about by rolling and squirming and may even creep and crawl. He will usually stand holding on when placed in that position and may well attempt to pull up to standing. Control in lowering is not well developed and it is always amusing to watch infants of this age drop back on to their well-padded rears.

Coincidental with this increased motor activity is the appearance of protective responses which increase the infant's safety. When he falls (or is made to fall) forwards or sideways, the arms or arm reflexively extend in a protective response.

Awareness of the surrounding world now extends beyond his mother's lap for several feet. He is aware of sounds in this extended environment and localizes them immediately and accurately. He visually searches the area and visually directs and controls his motor actions.

Examination at 9 months consists of:
Enquiry about parental concerns; progress and what the infant does now; use of hands; vocalizations.

Observation of activities, movements and vocalizations. When carried, needs little or no support of back and head. Note interaction between parent and child.

Measurements of weight and head circumference.

Examination of posture and activities in prone, sitting and supported upright positions. Note development of saving reactions.

With the child sitting comfortably offer 25 mm (1 in) cubes, first to one hand then the other – he should no longer take the cube with a palmar grasp but between thumb and fingers. When he has a cube in each hand, note if he compares them and knocks them together; when he has a cube in one hand, offer a second one and note the strategy used to deal with it. The developmental sequence is as follows:

ignores second cube; drops first cube and takes up second; attempts to take up second in the same hand; passes first cube to other hand and takes up second cube.

At 9 months one would expect to see one or both of the last two strategies.

Allow a cube to fall onto carpet or cloth (so no noise) and note if child looks for it. Allow child to see you cover the cube with a cloth or cup and note if he lifts up the cover to expose the cube.

Perform distraction test of hearing.

Note visual fixation and following, now possible at a greater distance – up to 3 m (10 ft). Disscreetly drop two or three 'hundreds and thousands' (cake decorations) onto a plain coloured cloth (e.g. green baize) and note visual fixation and fine pincer grasp.

Repeat cover test.

Note vocalizations and attempt to get vocal imitation.

Note reactions and behaviour.

12 months old (Figure 8.8)

The first birthday marks the end of a year of intensive progress which has brought the child to the stage of readiness for big advances in mobility and motor skills, language development, and exploration and domination of the world around.

One year olds like to be on their feet. Some will take a few steps with support, often with just one hand held, and a few are already walking independently. Pulling to stand and lowering down again, and cruising, are usually evident skills. Supine lying is now usually reserved for sleep, and an active infant in a supine position soon rises to sitting, or rolls to prone and then to crawling.

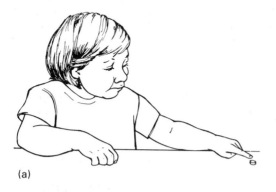
(a)

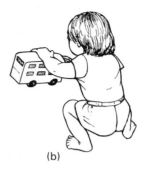
(b)

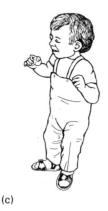
(c)

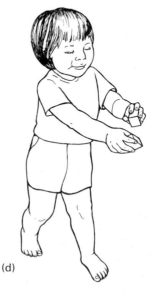
(d)

Figure 8.8 Twelve months old: (a) index approach well established; (b) squatting in play; (c) early steps (note posture of hands); (d) proferring cubes

Manipulative skills are now performed much more easily than at 9 months. The index finger is used for poking and pointing, objects are picked up between the thumb and finger, and the thumb–index pincer grip is neat and precise. Manipulative exploration and play occupy much of the daily activity. Simple objects such as blocks may be taken into each hand simultaneously and inspected, compared and knocked together. He shows great interest in playing give and take, searching for hidden objects, and pat-a-cake. He may recognize objects and will even attempt to use them for their correct purpose, for example, trying to feed himself with a spoon, to brush his hair, and to co-operate in dressing.

Visual exploration is well developed and manifest both with nearby objects and more distant surroundings. Auditory discrimination is developing, so enhancing interest in speech. His verbal understanding is exhibited by his behaviour in response to a few familiar words (e.g. daddy, dinner, walk). Learning is a very important part of his activities and clues to his ability in this respect come from seeing what use he makes of his newly acquired skills.

Examination at 12 months consists of:

Enquiry about parental concerns, motor activities, hand use and vocalizations.

Observation (a) of mobility, noting proficiency of crawling, cruising, pulling to stand and ability to take steps with support or alone; also note uses made of mobility.

(b) Of hand use – spontaneous manipulation, reaching, taking, giving. Note proficiency of finger–thumb opposition and use of index pointing,

(c) Of vocalizations, vocal imitation and play, and use for communication.

Measurement of weight and head circumference, and possibly length and blood pressure.

Examination (a) of play with cup and cube (putting in, taking out, seeking when hidden).

(b) Of reaction to everyday objects (e.g. cup, brush, spoon), and note attempts to use appropriately, thereby showing recognition of object.

(c) Of reactions to vocal play with imitation.

(d) Of visual ability and manipulation by noting response to small object, e.g. 'hundreds and thousands' or very small paper pellet.

Cover test may be repeated.

Interpretation of examinations in the first year

The purpose of the examinations is to confirm the absence of congenital malformations and the occurrence of satisfactory growth and development. The child should show an array of abilities appropriate for his age, of reasonable quality of performance and without abnormal features. Discrepancies of one or two features, or mild deviations, are not necessarily abnormal and may represent individual variation. Caution should be exercised before making firm diagnoses of deviation and abnormality. Experience and continued observation are both desirable requirements.

In the case of premature (pre-term) babies, the findings are related to a corrected age. For example, a baby born at 32 weeks' gestation with a chronological age of 5 months will have a corrected age of 3 months.

References

Atkinson, J. and Braddick, O. (1979) New techniques for assessing vision in infants and young children. *Child Care Hlth Dev.*, **5**, 389–398

Call, J. D. (1974) Helping infants cope with change. *Early Child Dev. Care,* **3**, 229–247

Catford, G. V. and Oliver, A. (1973) Development of visual acuity. *Arch. Dis. Childh.*, **48**, 47

Dobson, V. (1986) Assessment of visual acuity in infants and children. *Devl. Med. Child Neurol.*, **28**, 779–789

Hitchings, V. and Haggard, M. P. (1983) Incorporation of parental suspicions in screening infants. *Br. J. Audiol.*, **17**, 71–75

Mohn, D., Duin, J. H., Fetter, W. P. F., Groot, L. and Hage, M. (1988) Acuity card assessment of vision. *Devl. Med. Child Neurol.*, **30**, 232–244

Sheridan, M. D. (1973) The Stycar graded balls vision test. *Devl. Med. Child Neurol.*, **15**, 423

Teller, D. Y., McDonald, M. A., Preston, K., Sebris, S. L. and Dobson, V. (1986) Assessment of visual acuity in infants and children, the Acuity Card Procedure. *Devl. Med. Child Neurol.*, **28**, 779–789

Chapter 9

Development: 1–5 years

During the 4 years between their first and fifth birthday, children rapidly develop motor and language skills and use them to explore and to control their environment. There are so many new things to discover, and so much to do, that there is never a dull moment – life is activity or sleep. These activities enable them to wean themselves from close maternal attachment. Although all is 'child's play', adults still have an important role during these years.

The first independent steps of the 1 year old are the beginning of a rapid spurt of motor activity. Many new motor skills are acquired, including running, hopping, skipping, climbing, throwing, catching. With practice these are performed with greater and greater ease and precision, enabling the child to explore his environment which he does with great satisfaction. His environment widens and he feels himself to be the king of his domain. These activities open up possibilities for learning and opportunities for social play.

This is also the period in which children develop much understanding which is so distinctly human and so important for later intellectual development. They learn to understand the basic attributes of objects – their size, shape, weight, nature and colour. Add to this an ability to recognize similarities and differences between objects and they have the foundation for systems of classification and coding which contribute to later learning. Most important is the acquisition of ability to understand that objects can be represented by models, drawings and words. This whole process of symbolic representation and identification enhances the child's learning potential and means of communication.

The development of language during this period enables children to understand and to follow verbal messages and commands; to formulate their ideas and wishes; and to express themselves in speech. They use expressive language to tell of their experiences and wishes, and to control the activities of themselves and others. Language bears resemblances to mobility in that its acquisition widens their world, enhances social interaction and provides them with a tool with which they can control their world. The development of self-awareness and self-importance finds expression in their behaviour. Wider exploration of their surroundings and a growing awareness of others help them through this stage towards a willingness and desire for co-operative play with others. These transitions require many adjustments which are often accompanied by varied reactions. Much of this period may be spent in rebellion, but these problems are usually resolved as they approach 5 years of age.

Independence develops in many ways. The development of locomotor and manipulative skills makes each child independent, so far as choosing his own position and seeing to his own needs of washing, dressing and feeding are concerned. Personal independence also requires emancipation from parents and an ability to make a voluntary choice of friends in the group with which he identifies himself. The extensive development of these 4 years produces children who are ready to enter the wider world of school life. They are ready to take their first steps to be men and women of the world, but many years of training and development pass before this adult stage is reached.

The years from 1 to 5 are eventful in other respects. The children's environment expands and moves from the confines of the home to include the playgroup and nursery school. More siblings may appear in the family. Other children, both older and younger, and both from within the family and without, bring many interests to the developing children.

Table 9.1 summarizes the main features of development during this period.

Development of gross motor skills

By his first birthday an infant has well-established motor skills – he moves about and enjoys being on his feet. He is acquiring the abilities necessary for the development of motor skills, including:

(a) development of chain responses so that one movement leads into the next;
(b) acquisition of control of the speed and strength of the actions, and of the sequence and timing of the muscle actions to ensure smooth effective movements;
(c) awareness of the task involved;
(d) selection of the movements to carry out the task;
(e) selection of the muscle actions to perform the movements;
(f) awareness of different actions which can be used to achieve one particular task, and the choice of one of these;
(g) choice of whether and when to carry out the action.

The next few years are full of physical activity as he practises and perfects his motor skills and acquires new ones. The toddler seems to be on the go all the time. He loves to run, tumble, climb and fight. The following are a selection of the most common gross motor skills of early childhood (unless stated otherwise, the age levels refer to the age when 50% of normal children show the particular ability).

Walking
First independent steps appear at about 1 year of age. The upper acceptable limit is 18 months (Neligan and Prudham, 1969; Frankenberg *et al.*, 1971). At 18 months many children walk well, and some can walk backwards. Other walking skills include:

Walking on tiptoe: 2½ years.
Walking along a straight line (25 mm [1 in] wide, 3 m [10 ft] long):
    not more than 3 steps off: 2½ years;
    no steps off: 3 years.

Table 9.1 Summary of developmental progress, 1–5 yr

Age	Motor	Vision and manipulation	Hearing and language	Social
12–18 mth	Independent walking develops. Likes to push and pull wheeled toys. Often squats when playing. Climbs onto chairs. Goes up stairs usually with hand held and may attempt coming down, sometimes by bumping down on bottom	Enjoys picture books, points with finger. Much practice of eye–hand co-ordination. Sees small objects and picks them up with thumb and index finger. Does not yet turn book pages individually	Rapid development of vocabulary, especially of concrete nouns and verbs of action. Likes jingles. Understands single simple commands	Becoming independent in feeding. Aware of and disapproves of wetness. Plays alone, but needs adult nearby. Vulnerable in unsuitable environment
18–24 mth	Earlier motor skills more proficient. Beginning to attempt kicking and throwing ball. Shows better judgement of size and position of objects, e.g. chairs	Likes to scribble with pencil, imitates vertical stroke. Turns book pages singly	Beginning to join words. Echolalia often normally present. Carries out verbal requests	Responds to adult guidance and control. Not yet co-operative with peers, although may play alongside them. Domestic mimicry
2–3 yr	Very mobile, using this ability for exploration. Likes nursery climbing frame and large boxes to climb into and out of. Rides tricycle. Much more nimble. Walks sideways and backwards	Beginning of letter recognition which can be used in testing visual acuity. More mature hold of crayon. Copies circle. Beginning to thread beads and use scissors	Language well developed. May be expressed so quickly that intelligibility is reduced. Uses language for questioning and to direct actions. Repeats and sings nursery rhymes	Clings to mother. Often has favourite toy or rag. May rebel over feeding. Beginning to help with undressing and dressing. Will help with tidying away
3–4 yr	Now skilful in motor activities. Modifies speed and negotiates skilfully. Likes to try new skills, e.g. standing tiptoe, hopping	Beginning to make recognizable two-dimensional line drawings, e.g. house, man	Verbal skills and activities increased. Likes to hear and to relate long stories	Imaginative play in which everyday activities are imitated and children take adult roles. Tolerance of short separation and waiting developing. Beginning to share. Understanding good and bad
4–5 yr	Walks on straight line. Stands on one leg. Hops and skips with alternating feet. Responds to rhythm and music and movement. Group activities enjoyed	Hand skills developing rapidly. Colours pictures. Much neater and quicker	Fluent speech, free of infantile patterns	More confident and independent. May like to be 'king of the castle'. Likes small groups but group identity not strong. Play influenced by sex of child and culture

Walking along a circular line (25 mm [1 in] wide, 1.2 mm [4 ft] diameter):
  not more than 3 steps off: 3 years,
  no steps off: 4 years (McCaskill and Wellman, 1938).
Walking heel-toe: this ability appears early in the fourth year and is shown by 90%
of children by 5 years of age.

Running
This skill develops during the second year and is usually well established by the
second birthday.
  By 5 years of age all children should be able to run 30 yds (27 m) in under 10 s;
and by 9 years in under 7 s (Keogh, 1965).
  Timed standards for a 40-yard (36 m) sprint are shown in Table 9.2 (Arnheim and
Pestolesi, 1973).

Table 9.2 Timed standards for 40 yd (36 m) sprint (in seconds)

Percentage level	Age (yr)				
	5	6	7	8	9
50%	8.4	8.3	8.2	7.8	7.4
5% (assumed limit of acceptable normal)	9.7	9.5	9.4	9.2	8.9

Negotiating steps
There is very wide variation in acquiring this ability depending upon support,
method adopted, experience and confidence.
  Going up, without support, alternating feet: 2½ years.
  Going down, without support, alternating feet: 4 years (McCaskill and Wellman,
1938).

One-leg skills
The ability to stand on one leg appears at about 3 years of age. Mean duration of
maintenance of this posture is as follows:

3½ years: 2 s.
4 years: 4–8 s.
5 years: over 8 s.
Hopping on the spot: 5 times, 4 years; 10 times, 5 years (McCaskill and Wellman,
                      1938).
Hopping forwards: at 5 years, mean time for 50 ft (15 m), 10.5 s; at 10 years,
                      mean time for 50 ft, 4.8 s (Keogh, 1965).

Jumping
The first efforts at jumping often consist of stepping down or dropping from a step.
Such early jumping down a small distance is greatly affected by confidence. Most
children learn to lead with one foot at first and only later jump with both feet
together. The 50% age levels are as follows (McCaskill and Wellman, 1938):

Depth	One foot leading	Both feet together
12 in (0.3 m)	2 years	3 years
18 in (0.45 m)	2½ years	3 years

The standing jump is a complicated manoeuvre which begins with the child standing with his feet together and then by a sudden co-ordinated effort springing with both feet together to project the body forwards. Children acquire considerable ability, as shown by the distances they cover. In the later school years, boys do much better than girls, so the standards in these later years are shown separately for the two sexes in Table 9.3 (Arnheim and Pestolesi, 1973).

The minimal acceptable distance (i.e. 2 SD below mean) for a standing jump is 20 in (0.5 m) at 5 years and 43 in (1 m) at 10 years (Keogh, 1965).

Table 9.3 Fifty per cent and 5 per cent levels for standing jump (in inches)

Percentage level	Age (yr)				
	5	*6*	*7*	*8*	*9*
50%	37	40	43	47	53
5%	26	29	32	36	40
	10	*11*	*12*	*13*	*14*
50% (girls/boys)	55/60	58/62	60/66	60/70	63/76
5% (girls/boys)	42/48	45/48	45/48	45/53	46/59

Kicking

The ability to kick a ball forwards develops in the second year and is possessed by 90% of children by 2 years of age (Frankenberg *et al.*, 1971). The developmental stages of kicking are shown in Table 9.4.

Table 9.4 Developmental stages of kicking

	Stage			
	1	*2*	*3*	*4*
Age range (mth)	<12–36	12–78	18–>84	48–>84
Gaze	at ball	at ball	at ball	at ball and at target
Position	walks into ball	positions self for standing kick	runs to ball and kicks while running	as before but smoother
Kick (stationary ball)	none	leg flexed at hip	knee also flexed, then extended to give good kick	as before but smoother
Moving ball	none	none	none	anticipates and kicks moving ball

Catching and throwing

A child's behaviour with a ball reveals much about manipulative ability, and in addition shows the importance of timing and perceptual awareness of the task. Kay's (1970) description of all the events involved in catching a ball is particularly lucid and should be read by all who study this subject. The 50% levels (i.e. the age at which 50% of children are able to achieve that level of performance) for various ball abilities are shown in Table 9.5 (McCaskill and Wellman, 1938).

Table 9.5 Fifty per cent age levels for certain ball skills of children

Bounce along with one hand a distance of:	3 ft	2 yr
	5 ft	3½ yr
Catch with arms straight		3 yr
Catch with arms bent		4 yr
Throw with one hand a distance of:	5 ft	2½ yr
	10 ft	4 yr
	15 ft	5½ yr

Table 9.6 Variability of ball skills according to age and sex

	Age and sex			
	5 yr		10 yr	
	Male	Female	Male	Female
Distance thrown (in ft), mean	34	19	94	49
2 SD mean (assumed as the minimal acceptable normal level)	22	4	52	13

Ball-throwing skill varies greatly between children. At each age there is a wide range on either side of the mean, and there are also marked sex differences, as shown in Table 9.6 (Keogh, 1965).

The developmental stages of catching (Table 9.7) show the importance of visual adjustment, anticipation of the task, timing of actions and smoothness of performance.

The developmental stages of throwing (Table 9.8) show the importance of body poise, involvement of different arm joints and timing, especially with regard to release of the ball.

After the first year many other motor skills appear and then become increasingly developed, as shown by increased speed and precision and decreased effort in performance. Some skills show a similar pattern of development and proficiency in both boys and girls, e.g. a short run (Figure 9.1). Boys tend to be superior even from the early years in skills involving strength, e.g. throwing a ball (Table 9.6), whereas girls are superior in skills involving precision, e.g. mat-hopping test (Figure 9.2).

Table 9.7 Developmental stages of catching

	Stage				
	1	*2*	*3*	*4*	*5*
Age range (mth)	12–42	24–60	24–>84	48–>84	54–>84
Gaze	ahead at thrower	at ball in thrown hands	at own hands and approaching ball	follows flight of ball	as before but better
Arm	neutral, no preparation	extended	elbows flexed, hands cupped, early anticipation	arms flexed and move to anticipate ball	as before but more relaxed
Reactions	none, or arches back and stretches arms	traps ball in flexed arms against chest	catches ball in hands	catches direct throw easily and to the side sometimes	smooth movements
Success	none	about 50%	100%	direct 100%, side about 50%	100%

Table 9.8 Developmental stages of throwing

	Stage				
	1	*2*	*3*	*4*	*5*
Age range (mth)	12–36	12–54	18–72	30–84	36–>84
Arms	crude attempt using one or both arms	one arm used, kept extended, movement only at shoulder	either arm used, sudden flexion of elbow now seen	preferred arm used; wrist flexion now seen	preferred arm used; finger movements now as well as movement at shoulder, elbow and wrist
Trunk	no particular position	no particular position	tends to lean forwards	trunk moves with throw	arches back and moves forwards with throw
Legs	no particular stance	no particular stance	one leg advanced	one leg advanced	one leg advanced, good poise
Release	erratic	erratic	controlled dropping	dropping now, more a throw	thrown with good timing
Distance	very little	a yard or two	increasing	increasing	quite considerable
Accuracy	nil	very little	same	fairly good	good

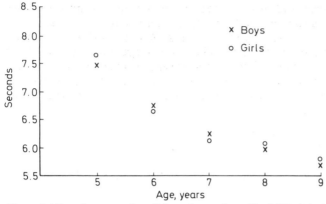

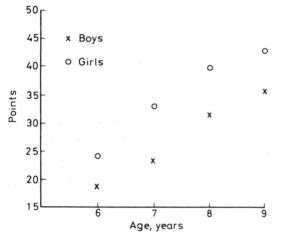

Figure 9.1 Development of proficiency in running – 30 yd (27 m) dash; mean scores, age 5–9 (Keogh, 1965)

Figure 9.2 Girls' superiority over boys in precision skill – mat-hopping test; mean scores, age 6–9 (Keogh, 1965)

Development of hand skills

Study of the evolution of manipulative skills requires an analysis of all the mechanisms involved and consideration of the significance of the actions. The principal items are as follows:

(a) maturation of neuromuscular actions;
(b) increase of speed and precision;
(c) development of new perceptual awareness;
(d) development of new skills.

Manipulation of cubes

Building a tower of cubes requires considerable perceptual ability. The child has to be aware of the task, to be able to follow the demonstration, and to have the manipulative skill to carry it out. Some babies at 1 year of age understand what is required and make an attempt, but few succeed. Success comes a month or two later, and from then onwards they are able to build a higher tower at successive ages: 3 cubes at 1½ years, 6 at 2 years, and 9 at 3 years. With regard to this action, no new learning is involved during this time. The test is largely a measure of the child's manipulative ability, combined with perceptual awareness of the task involved which was present from early in the second year. It is interesting to note the variations of the normal expectations in the test as quoted by different authors. At the age of 2 years a tower of:

2 or more cubes (Buchler and Hetzer, 1935; Stutsman, 1948);
4 cubes (Terman and Merrill, 1937; Valentine, 1985);
5 cubes (Griffiths, 1954);
6–7 cubes (Gesell and Amatruda, 1947; Illingworth, 1966; Sheridan, 1960; Slosson, 1963; Bayley, 1965).

These authors differ not only with respect to their expectations in these tests, but also in the way in which they are performed. For example, in the Merrill–Palmer test the child is expected to add two more cubes to a tower started by the examiner, or to build a three-cube tower from the beginning. The Stanford–Binet test requirement of a four or more cube tower is in imitation of the examiner's, whereas the Griffith's test five-cube tower is not so.

These simple examples show how much can be learnt from observing children building towers of cubes, and also that reliance upon a precise score in a test may be misleading unless the test and its method of administration are fully understood by the examiner. More complex tasks with cubes explore both perceptual abilities as well as manipulative skills. In some tests the child is asked to complete a particular task and is allowed unlimited time, but in others his performance is timed, or the task has to be completed within a time limit.

Examples are as follows. (N.B. This list is not compiled as a test. These examples should suffice to show how they can be used to explore various aspects of motor perception and skill.)

Aligns 2 or more cubes as a 'train' (2 years, Gesell).

Aligns 3 or more cubes as a 'train' (2½ years, Bayley).

Adds 'chimney' to train (2½ years, Gesell).

Builds a pyramid from 3 cubes in:

17 s (3 years), 11 s (3½ years), 9 s (4 years), 7 s (4½ years) (Merrill–Palmer).

Builds a pyramid from 6 cubes in:

35 s (4½ years), 20 s (5 years) (Merrill–Palmer).

Builds bridge by imitation (i.e. child watches it being done and then does it himself) (3 years) and from model (i.e. child is shown completed item (3½ years) (Gesell).

Builds gate by imitation (4 years) and from model (4½ years) (Gesell).

Manipulation of pencil and paper

Another aspect of manipulative skill which can be studied with advantage is a child's performance with pencil and paper. Several aspects will be considered.

Handling pencil and paper

Given an opportunity, children soon show an interest in using a pencil and paper in imitation of older children and adults. At first the grip upon the pencil is a cylindrical one, with the pencil being treated rather like a rod (Figure 9.3). The

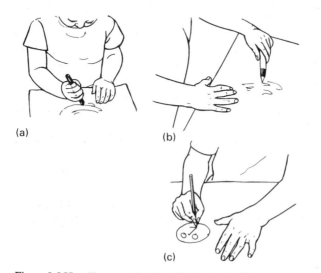

Figure 9.3 Handling pencils: (a) cylindrical grip; (b) early thumb–finger grip; (c) dynamic tripod

point projects from the lower, ulnar border of the hand and scribbling marks are made with a stirring-like action. If the pencil is taken into the hand the other way up, the child sometimes realizes that he can use it by pronating the forearm and so bringing the point into contact with the paper. Usually at this early stage the child can do no more than scribble. This limitation is due mostly to immaturity and is not due just to the type of grip, because more perceptually advanced children are seen sometimes who, for one reason or another, retain this immature grip pattern, but are able, nevertheless, to make accurate reproductions on paper.

A big step forwards comes when the pencil is held between the thumb and fingers, especially the first two fingers. The fingers are usually held stiffly at first and only later do they relax so that a mature grip can occur. This mature grip is called the dynamic tripod in order to emphasize that three digits are involved together (thumb, index finger and middle finger), and that they are constantly moving to adjust the position of the pencil.

Handedness

Handedness is a complex subject which is discussed only briefly here. Children usually begin to show a preference for using one hand rather than the other during their second year. As this preference becomes established, it may be so well marked in some children that there is no doubt that they are right- or left-handed. In other cases the preference is not so marked, and in the early years, at least, they may alternate from time to time.

Much has been written, often rather uncritically, about the implications of ill-defined hand preference and its relationship to cerebral dominance, neurological disturbance and learning difficulties. A more sceptical attitude to some of these sweeping assertions is needed and a critical review of this topic by Touwen (1972) is especially useful.

At the present time there are several generalizations which are widely accepted:

1. Any child showing extremely strong preference for one hand may have some neurological deficits of the other side.
2. Left-handed children have to make more adjustments than right-handed children because everyday articles are arranged for right-handed users, e.g. door handles. Also, writing from left to right across a page is easier for right-handed than for left-handed children. When writing with the left hand, the writing already on the sheet is obscured by the hand unless, as often happens, some unusual posture is adopted. Barsley (1966) described the problems encountered by left-handed people very vividly.
3. Among children with uncertain and mixed preferences there is a greater than average number with neurological disturbances.
4. It is dangerous to attribute a child's difficulties to handedness problems without very careful evaluation.

Preferred handedness, footedness and eyeness can be determined by simple tests, as listed in Table 9.9. Although these are simple tests, care is required in

Table 9.9 Tests for hand, foot and eye preference

Handedness	Footedness	Eyeness
Pick up a pencil to write	Kick a ball	Look into a telescope held for him
Put a small object in a box	Tap a tune with a foot	Align a gun on target
Press a bell-push	Squash a small object with a foot	Examine a suitable object, e.g. postage stamp, with a magnifying lens held for him

order to avoid misleading results. For example, the objects for the child to pick up must be placed before him in the mid-line, and objects for the child to look into or through must be held for him; otherwise, if the child is allowed to take it up himself, he will do so with his preferred hand and will then be more likely to use the eye on that side because it is easier to do so whether or not it is the preferred eye. Also, whenever eyeness is being tested, it is important to ensure that visual function is equal on the two sides. Obviously, differences in visual function will affect eye preference, yet there have been scores of reports on laterality and crossed laterality which have ignored this point. More complicated tests exist for a full investigation of laterality such as those described by Benton (1959).

Imitating and copying symbols

Most children love to play with pencil and paper, and observing whether or not they can reproduce various symbols gives information about their perceptual awareness. Ability to draw straight lines running horizontally, vertically and obliquely, lines joining and crossing, areas enclosed by circles and by angulated figures and so forth are examined in many of the psychological tests for young children. In the performance and scoring of these tests, a clear distinction must be made between *imitation*, i.e. the child draws the symbol after seeing the examiner do so, and *copying*, i.e. the child draws the symbol from a picture of the completed symbol which is placed in front of him either throughout, or for a set period before he is asked to draw. A definite developmental sequence is seen in the reproduction of symbols and this is summarized in Table 9.10. This table is not meant to represent a test, but to show the developmental sequence.

Table 9.10 Developmental sequence of symbol imitation and copying

Symbol	Description	Approximate age level (yr)	
		Imitation	Copy
/	Stroke – random	1½	–
|	Stroke – horizontal or vertical	2	2½
○	Circle	2	3
+	Cross	3	3½–4
□	Square	3½–4	4½
△	Triangle	4–4½	5

When these abilities are examined in tests, definite criteria are laid down concerning the manner of presentation of task, the number of attempts which are permissible and whether or not the symbol produced can be accepted.

Drawing

Children's drawings reflect their draughtsmanship, perceptual awareness, knowledge and understanding of the world around them, and their personal feelings (Harris, 1963; Di Leo, 1967). They are a rich source of exploration for any student of child development and behaviour. A child's awareness of body parts and their relationship is brought out in the Goodenough Draw-a-Man test (Goodenough, 1926). The child is asked to draw a person and is given all the time he requires to do so. He may be prompted to make sure that he has included everything. Then one point is awarded for each of the items of the drawing which is on the list below (no half points).

1. Head present – any clear method of representing the head.
2. Legs present – any method of presentation clearly intended to indicate legs. Number must be correct for the position.
3. Arms present – any method of representation clearly intended to indicate arms. Fingers alone not sufficient – credit if any space left between base of fingers and body where attached. Number must be correct.
4. (a) Trunk present – any clear indication of trunk, whether by straight line only, or by some sort of two-dimensional figure.
   (b) Length of trunk greater than breadth – measurement should be taken at points of greatest length and breadth. If equal score minus.
   (c) Shoulders definitely indicated – ordinary elliptical form never credited, score minus if trunk square or rectangular.
5. (a) Attachment of arms and legs – both arms and legs attached at any point, or arms to neck, or at junction of head and trunk.
   (b) Legs attached to the trunk. Arms attached to trunk at correct point. If 4(c) plus, point of attachment must be exactly at shoulders. If 4(c) minus, attachment must be exactly at point where shoulders should have been indicated.
6. (a) Neck present – any clear indication.
   (b) Outline of neck continuous with that of hand, or trunk, or of both.
7. (a) Eyes present – either one or both.
   (b) Nose present – any clear method of representation.
   (c) Mouth present – any clear method.
   (d) Both nose and mouth shown in two dimensions – two lips shown.
   (e) Nostrils shown – any clear method.
8. (a) Hair shown – any clear method.
   (b) Hair present over more than the circumference of the head. Better than a scribble. Non-transparent, i.e. outline of head not showing through the hair.
9. (a) Clothing present – any clear method, e.g. buttons.
   (b) At least two articles of clothing (as hat and trousers), non-transparent, i.e. concealing part of body supposed to cover.
   (c) Entire drawing free from transparencies of any sort. Both sleeves and trousers must be shown.
   (d) At least four articles of clothing definitely indicated – hat, coat, shirt, collar, tie, belt or braces, trousers.
   (e) Costume complete without incongruities – a definite and recognizable kind of costume, e.g. suit. No confusion permitted. Hat must always be shown if part of costume, e.g. uniform. Sleeves and trousers must be shown, also shoes.
10. (a) Fingers present – any clear indication.
    (b) Correct number of fingers shown – five or 10, according to hands shown.
    (c) Details of fingers correct, two dimensions, length greater than breadth; and the angle subtended by them not greater than 180°.
    (d) Opposition of thumb shown – any clear differentiation from fingers.
    (e) Hand shown as distinct from fingers and arms.

11. (a) Arm joint shown – either elbow, shoulder or both – curve only at elbow, score minus.
    (b) Leg joint shown – either knee, hip or both – abrupt bend for knee. Hip, if inner lines of legs meet at point of junction with body, credited.
12. (a) Proportion. Head – area not more than half or less than one-tenth of trunk. Score rather leniently.
    (b) Proportion. Arms – equal to trunk in length or slightly longer, but not reaching knees. Width of legs less than trunk.
    (c) Proportion. Legs – length not less than vertical measurement of trunk, nor greater than twice that. Width of legs less than trunk.
    (d) Proportion. Feet – feet and legs must be shown in two dimensions. Length of foot must be greater than height from sole to instep. Length of foot not more than one-third or less than one-tenth total length of leg. Credited on full-face if shown in perspective, provided foot separated in some way from rest of leg.
    (e) Proportion. Two dimensions. Both arms and legs shown in two dimensions.
13. Heel shown – any clear method. Credited on full-face drawings where foot is shown in perspective.
14. (a) Motor co-ordination. Lines A. All lines reasonably firm, meeting each other clearly. Degree of complexity of drawing to be taken into account – if few lines score more severely.
    (b) Motor co-ordination. Lines B. All lines firmly drawn with correct jointing. Score very strictly.
    (c) Motor co-ordination. Head outline – outline of head without obviously unintentional irregularities. Simple ellipse not credited.
    (d) Motor co-ordination. Trunk outline – as for (c).
    (e) Motor co-ordination. Arms and legs without irregularities and without tendency to narrowing at junction with body. Arms and legs in two dimensions.
    (f) Motor co-ordination. Features symmetrical in all respects – eyes, nose, mouth in two dimensions. Score strictly. More likely to be plus if profile rather than full-face.
15. (a) Ears present – one or two according to profile or full-face. Any clear method.
    (b) Ears present in correct position and proportion – vertical measurement must be greater than horizontal. In profile, some detail for aural canal. Within middle of two-thirds of head.
16. (a) Eye detail – brow, lashes or both shown. Any clear method.
    (b) Eye detail – pupil shown. Dot with curved line above not credited, as dot represents eye itself and is credited in 7(a).
    (c) Eye detail – proportion. Horizontal measurement of eye must be greater than vertical.
    (d) Eye detail – glance. Face must be in profile. Eye shown either in perspective or, if almond form, pupil must be placed towards front of eye rather than in centre.
17. (a) Both chin and forehead shown – eyes and mouth present, sufficient space left for chin and forehead. Score rather leniently.
    (b) Projection of chin shown, chin clearly differentiated from lower lip.

18. (a) Head, trunk and feet shown in profile without error. One only of these errors allowed: bodily transparency, legs not in profile, arms attached to outline of back and extending forward.
    (b) Figure shown in true profile, without error of bodily transparency, except that shape of eye may be ignored.

Each point credited is the equivalent of a quarter of a year. To calculate the mental age, count the total number of points scored and divide this by 4. Add 3 to the result. This gives the mental age in years (3 years is credited as this is immediately below the age level at which the scoring begins). Forty points gives a mental age of 13 years. The scale is not valid beyond this, although the maximum score on the test is 51 points (Goodenough, 1926) (Figure 9.4).

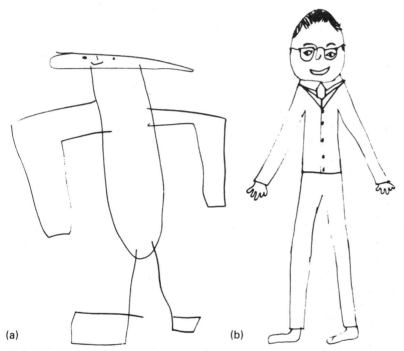

(a)   (b)

Figure 9.4 Goodenough Draw-a-Man test: (a) drawing by boy aged 7 years with a mental age of 7 years; (b) drawing by boy aged 8 years with a mental age of 11½ years

Observing a child's drawing of a house reveals his awareness of spatial relationships and of perspective. Free drawings, especially if accompanied by discussion with the child, provide much information about conceptual and emotional development which is beyond the scope of this volume. The interested reader is referred to other literature on this subject (Bender, 1938; Harris, 1963; Di Leo, 1967).

Further manipulative skills

Tea-set play
Doll's tea-set play reveals the development of a young child's manipulative ability particularly well. This is a fascinating task for a 2–5-year-old child and is seldom

associated with any difficulties of administration. Horton and Rosenbloom (1971) used this technique to study manipulative skill in young children. They analysed the movements and efforts involved in the task. While children play with the tea-set, observations are concentrated upon the teapot and note is made of how the child holds and controls it in pouring, the adjustment of height of pouring, appreciation of degree of filling of the cup and overall precision and freedom from spilling (Figure 9.5). This method is not a standardized test, but a definite sequence occurs

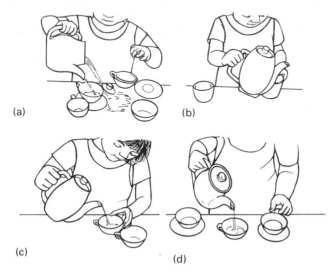

(a)

(b)

(c)

(d)

Figure 9.5 Doll's tea-set play: (a) early stage, cylindrical grip, poor positioning and spilling; (b) positioning still imprecise; (c) hand rotated to give better control; (d) precise positioning and pouring

in the development of skill in handling the teapot, and it is possible to indicate approximate age levels for the different stages, as follows:

1. Holds teapot handle with a cylindrical grip and may steady it with other hand; attempts to pour without lifting teapot or only lifting part way; frequently spilling occurs – around 2½–3 years of age.
2. Holds teapot handle with a cylindrical grip; raises teapot to pour, but height and position in relation to cup may be ill-judged and frequent spilling occurs – around 3–3½ years of age.
3. Holds teapot handle with a cylindrical grip and with hand rotated so as to permit control of the teapot by radio-ulnar movement at the wrist; much better judgement of distances and of filling of cup; little spilling occurs – around 3½–4 years of age.
4. Teapot handle held with a cylindrical grip as before and also with thumb on spine of handle to give better control in pouring, which is now more precise and there is no spilling – around 4–4½ years of age.

Pegs and cup manipulation

Some years ago I described a simple test of manipulation which has proved very useful in clinical practice (Holt, 1965). A child of 1 year can pick up a small peg and drop it into a cup. Although the task is understood at this early age, the performance is very imperfect. Performance improves steadily with age, and up to 10 years of age the relationship between speed of performance and age is virtually linear, so it is possible to devise tests based upon age norms.

In the tests the child is asked to pick up pegs one at a time and to drop them into a cup as quickly as he can. The best score in three tries over a set time – usually 30 s – is noted. The child is then asked to take up pegs one at a time and to place them in a peg board. The best score in three tries – in the same time – is noted. The results in both these tests are related to age. The score on the second test is directly dependent upon the score of the first test; thus, by knowing the child's age and score on the first test, it is possible to predict the score which should be obtained on the second test (Figure 9.6). An actual score appreciably below that predicted indicates impairment of manipulation. This test enables one to examine manipulative ability without confusion from intellectual influences.

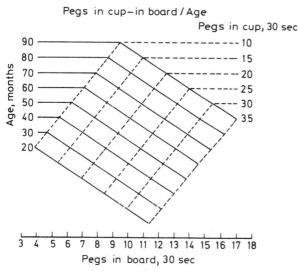

Figure 9.6 Manipulation tests – pegs and cup. Prediction of score on board test from age and score in cup test. Example, a child aged 60 months who puts 20 pegs in cup would be expected to put 10 into the board

Other abilities

By 5 years of age a child possesses a wide range of arm and hand skills which he can use in many ways, ranging from dressing to drawing.

Touching and reaching – the extended arm moving at the shoulder covers a wide area and the range is increased by leaning forwards or sideways, standing on toes or squatting.

Taking hold of and examining – the arm reaches out, objects are taken into the hand and then brought to the mouth for eating or close to the eyes for examination or passed to the other hand. The actions performed by the hand and fingers include the following:

index finger pointing; thumb pressing; spreading fingers to open up something; thumb used in opposition to index finger as in fine pick-up, and against other fingers in a cylindrical grasp.

Movements at the wrist permit a variety of grips to be performed. The actions used to perform screwing movements vary according to the magnitude of the task. Large rotatory screwing actions require movement at the shoulder; lesser ones involve pronation and supination of the forearm; and very fine ones are performed by rolling actions between the finger tips.

The arms can be used together in a bear-like hug or to lift a heavy object. Often one hand acts as assistant to the other, but each hand can be used to execute most complex activities simultaneously, as in piano playing.

Sensory development

The physiological bases for sensory functions were well established in the first year, so that by 1 year of age a child can hear acutely and locate the source of sounds, has well-developed peripheral and central vision and can converge and accommodate. During this period there occurs development of recognition of what is seen and heard.

The child learns to listen and to recognize more sounds, as described below in the development of receptive language.

The development of visual recognition proceeds from three-dimensional objects to three-dimensional models to two-dimensional pictures and to symbols. Simple geometric symbols such as vertical and horizontal lines are recognized first, then enclosed figures such as a circle or square and then increasingly complex ones. The Stycar vision tests for young children, devised by Sheridan (1969), incorporate this developmental sequence.

The links between sensory and other functions improve during this period, as is especially well seen in hand–eye activities.

Development of language

Human behaviour consists of the responses to internal and external stimuli. During the course of development the child becomes aware of many stimuli; he acquires

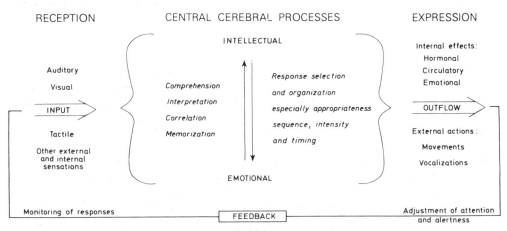

Figure 9.7 Central cerebral processes concerned with language

abilities to interpret and understand these stimuli, to select the important and useful ones, and to suppress or reject others. At the same time as the child responds to various stimuli, he notes the results of such responses. As development proceeds, his abilities to receive and to respond become more complex and more effective. Between these two aspects – the reception of stimuli and the performance of actions – are interposed the all-important cerebral mechanisms. They are alerted to receive various stimuli, to interpret and memorize the incoming sensations, and then to select an appropriate response and initiate the action (Figure 9.7).

Language development consists of the maturation of the central processes and simultaneous advancement of reception and expression (Figure 9.8).

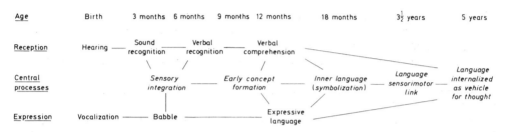

Figure 9.8 Diagrammatic representation of language development (Reynell, 1969)

The central language processes are not directly observable as are the receptive and expressive aspects. They can be revealed, however, by specially designed tests and by study of language disorders in children.

Reception

Infants begin to give more attention to sounds they hear frequently, clearly and in association with other pleasurable sensations. The infant learns to recognize sounds he makes himself to distinguish them from those made in other ways. He then begins to recognize and understand words. The observation of these changes reflects the integrative processes in the brain and the associated cognitive development.

Expression

Some expressions have an immediate effect upon the environment, e.g. a shrill cry in a moment of temper, but other expressions are only effective if they are received, accepted and interpreted by another person, and this is the basis of interpersonal communication. Expressions may be divided into those which are (a) deliberately communicative, (b) coincidently communicative, and (c) non-communicative.

The process of communication can be extremely complex and sophisticated, according to the subtlety of the expressions and the ingenuity and sensitivity of the observer. Expressions based upon movements and actions are often fairly crude, but facial expressions and eye movements can be used to convey a wide range of meanings. Indeed, a glance between two people may convey a world of meaning which could not be communicated as effectively in any other way. An astounding degree of communication is sometimes achieved between severely disabled children and their mothers. Other attendants may find the same child completely unresponsive because: (a) they do not create an environment which encourages attempts at expression and communication by the handicapped child; (b) they do not recognize the expressions used by the child for communication; and (c) they do not have the mental preparedness to accept and interpret the expressions. In any of these circumstances, communication never begins or soon fails through lack of reinforcement.

Some individuals communicate by expressions known only to themselves. Twins, for example, appear to anticipate each other's wishes and actions by means of expressions to which they are particularly sensitive, but which are seldom apparent to others.

Expressions can be divided into vocal and non-vocal groups. The above examples of communication were mostly non-vocal. Vocal expressions cover a wide range of situations and may be used for many purposes. They are particularly useful for communication at a distance. An extension and elaboration of vocal expression is available to humans in the form of verbal expression. Expressive language consists of the externalization of inner language produced by the central cerebral processes.

Verbalization

Verbalization develops when vocalizations are modified to reproduce word sounds. An ability to select and imitate sounds is important for verbalization to develop. Constant repetition is necessary. It has been estimated that infants are usually exposed to 500–600 repetitions of a word before they reproduce it. The spoken word, unlike the written word, is gone once it has been uttered and cannot be referred back to. Even so, the imitation of familiar speech sounds does not at first constitute expressive language. It has to be linked with the recognition of the objects being named and the realization that they can be identified by a sound, a word, a name. The central process which bring about this recognition and realization are normally developing while the infants are learning to be aware of sounds and to imitate them.

The processes involved in the development of speech will be better understood by considering a particular example; for instance, an infant learning to recognize, identify and name his own cup (Table 9.11). Several times a day, as he sits on his mother's lap or in his high-chair with her nearby, he will be given pleasurable drinks from the same container. He will hear many times his mother refer to his 'cup' and will learn to associate this word with the object from which he has pleasurable drinks. The close proximity of his mother, the constant repetition at

Table 9.11 Processes involved in learning to recognize a cup

Child sees the cup on the table or in his mother's hand, begins to recognize shape

Child touches the cup, lifts it and bangs it, begins to recognize the feel of it

Child hears his mother say 'cup' as she holds it or gives him a drink from it; begins to associate sound with object

Child enjoys drink from cup, begins to associate pleasurable experience with object and sound of word 'cup'

appropriate moments of the word 'cup', the recognition of his own cup and his ability to see it, touch it and take it to his mouth, all reinforce his learning of the word 'cup'. At first he may confuse the word for the container 'cup' with that for the contents 'milk'. Later on he will learn that there are other cups in addition to his own, and that cups are identifiable by their shape and the use to which they are put.

Most infants receive adequate verbal stimulation, but some do not. Some of the results of a study by Rheingold (1960), shown in Table 9.12, show how infants in an institutional nursery suffer as a result of inadequate verbal stimulation.

Table 9.12 Verbal stimulation in an institutional nursery as compared with home (Rheingold, 1960)

Item	Mean score	
	Home	Institution
Looks at infant's face	140	28
Talks to infant	166	17
Holds infant	285	46
Infant out of own room	304	43
1 or more adults within 6 ft (2 m)	524	217
Bottle in mouth	54	299

Children may develop an ability to imitate speech without acquiring the associated verbal concepts (and some, alas, are even trained to do so). At this early stage in the development of language, the acquisition of verbalization without the basic concepts has disastrous consequences. The problem is seen principally in children with cerebral disorders. Some retarded children who have not acquired this all-important central understanding of the meaning of the words they reproduce show repetitive word imitation (echolalia) which may continue for years without any progress in language development.

Difficulties in the accurate reproduction of word sounds, despite the acquisition of the appropriate concepts, occur quite commonly and usually are not serious. For example, one little girl knew her sister and her name 'Alison', but could not reproduce it exactly and called her 'Ice-on'. This was a temporary phase, however. Such discrepancies between concept readiness and quality of expressive language often occur in bright children whose thoughts seem to run ahead of their articulatory skills. This problem is sometimes seen even more markedly a year or two later when a child produces a long stream of unintelligible speech which often represents the outflow of many active ideas. The term *jargon* is used to describe unintelligible speech of this nature. In the situation quoted, the jargon was meaningful in that there were sensible ideas behind it, but sometimes jargon is meaningless.

Once verbalization has begun, it usually proceeds rapidly. In consequence, the average number of words produced at different ages increases sharply, as is shown in Table 9.13. The ability to identify an object which he can see and touch (a so-called concrete object) with a verbal label is a great achievement, and is one which the child applies to everything he encounters. This process normally occurs during his second year, and as a result he adds many nouns to his vocabulary at this time. He then begins to learn the verbal labels for actions he performs, such as drinking, sitting, walking, etc. His vocabulary then expands to include verbs of

Table 9.13 Size and type of vocabulary according to age (Duffy and Irwin, 1951)

Item	Age (yr)				
	1	2	3	4	5
Number of words	1–2	20–100	900	1500	>2000
Type of words:					
nouns	+	+	+	+	+
verbs		±	+	+	+
pronouns		±	+	+	+
adjectives			±	+	+
Sentence length		2–3 words	3–4 words		>5 words
Intelligibility		66%	90%		100%

action. The process of conceptualization and naming continues and his vocabulary expands rapidly. Because the child is becoming more aware of himself and of his relationships to others, there are frequent confusions of expression between 'I', 'me' and 'you', but these resolve in time. Later still he develops an ability to conceptualize abstract subjects and to name them. The great increase of expressive vocabulary with its sequence of nouns, verbs, personal pronouns and adjectives, is an outward manifestation of the increase in understanding which is occurring in the brain.

A big step forward occurs when the child becomes able to link concepts together. For example, 'Daddy gone' represents two clear concepts. 'Me ride it' indicates three concepts. A phrase like 'All gone', however, does not represent an advance, because although we see it as two distinct words and appreciate the meaning of 'all', to the young child the concept of 'all' is too abstract for him to understand as yet, and the phrase is really a double-syllabic single-concept one which represents no major advance upon 'gone' so far as language is concerned.

Symbolization

So far the discussion of the development of language has been concerned with the acquisition of vocabulary and the demonstration of the importance of the central processes of concept formation and association. There is another major process involved in the development of language, namely *symbolization*. Reynell (1969) described the development of symbolization very clearly, as: the process by which objects, persons, actions, and states are represented by some means which can be recognized intellectually by others. The simplest symbols are models or pictures of the real object. Verbal symbols are the spoken or written words which represent and identify the object.

A communication is symbolic when the content of the message is coded into symbols. Reynell defines language as *any* symbolic communication, and verbal language as communication by verbal symbols, i.e. words.

The linking of a name to the concept of an object is an early example of verbal symbolization and it greatly facilitates the development of both language and the acquisition of vocabulary. Not only does the process of symbolization promote the development of verbal language, it also facilitates the integration of the central processes concerned with reception and expression. For example, a cup may be represented symbolically by a model, picture, word or sign (Figure 9.9). The use of such symbols facilitates the integration of the visual, auditory and tactile impressions which arise from them. Through symbolization a child can take a picture, model, sign or other representation and not only recognize it as representing the real thing, but do to it what he might do to the real thing. Thus, a child might take a doll and play with it as if it were a baby, trying to feed, bathe and dress it. Much of a child's symbolic understanding is best seen in his play, and play observation forms an essential part of the evaluation of language development.

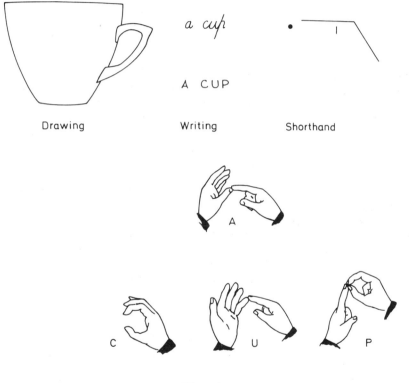

Figure 9.9 Symbolization: representation of 'a cup'

Observation of play is necessary for another purpose, namely, to observe the use of language in the direction of play. Young children often talk as they play. They are directing their own actions in this way until these actions have been fully internalized. Language plays an important part in the pre-school years when children use it to organize and integrate their actions. At this stage they can be helped by being guided in the sequencing of their actions.

The development of receptive and expressive language is summarized in Table 9.14, prepared by Sheridan (1975a). A programme to assist early language development is described by Cooper, Moodley and Reynell (1983).

Table 9.14 Outline of expected ages and stages in development of spoken language (Sheridan, 1975a)

Ages	Manifestations	Stages
4½ mth	Reception	Pays obvious attention to nearby meaningful sounds, particularly familiar voices
	Expression	Vocalizes responsively when spoken to face-to-face; chuckles and squeals. Babbles to self and others using sing-song intonation and single or double 'syllables'. Cries loudly when hungry, annoyed or uncomfortable
7 mth	Reception	Immediately attends to and localizes nearby everyday meaningful sounds, particularly human voices. Beginning to respond discriminately to emotional overtones in speech of familiar adults (e.g. soothing, prohibitive)
	Expression	Babbles continuously to self and others in long, tuneful repetitive strings of syllables with wide range of pitch, combining open vowels and (usually) single consonant sounds. Beginning to imitate adults' playful vocalizations in face-to-face situations
14 mth	Reception	Responds appropriately to quiet meaningful everyday sounds within 3 or 4 m. Recognizes own and family names and words for several common objects and activities. Sensitive to expressive cadences in speech of familiars
	Expression	Jabbers continuously to self and others employing loud, prosodic tuneful jargon. Emergence of first single words used correctly, consistently and spontaneously (i.e. not imitatively) but usually comprehensible, even to familiars, only in situational context. Ekes out articulatory difficulties with urgent intonations and finger pointings
21 mth	Reception	Shows clearly by correct response to spoken communications that he hears and understands many more words than he can utter
	Expression	Speaks 20 or 50+ single words and is beginning to join two or three words in meaningful sentences of agent–action–object type. Refers to self by name. Owing to numerous infantilisms, speech sometimes unintelligible to familiars and almost always to strangers. Echoes final or stressed word in sentences addressed to him. Shows brief imitative role-play alone or with friendly adult. Beginning to play meaningfully with miniature toys, accompanied by occasional spoken words
3 yr	Reception	Comprehends literal meanings of words and beginning to appreciate common semantic variations
	Expression	Echolalia persists. Vocabulary rapidly enlarging. Uses sentences of 3–5 words, personal pronouns and most prepositions. Talks continuously to self at play. Infantilisms of articulation and grammar gradually diminishing. Intelligible even to strangers. Asks many questions of who? what? where? type. Engages in simple make-believe play alone or with one or two others. Plays meaningfully with miniature toys, providing simultaneous running commentary
4½ yr	Reception	Competent for most everyday situations provided sentences are not longer than 6 or 7 words and vocabulary employed reflects child's experience
	Expression	Uses large vocabulary with conventional grammar and syntax. Articulation still shows residual infantilisms, chiefly involving r-l-w-y, t-k, and s-f-th consonant groups, but speech (usually) intelligible even to strangers. Narrates long stories. Asks numerous questions of when? why? how? type, and meanings of words. Engages in elaborate make-believe play with group of three to six peers. Draws 'pictures' (usually) of people, houses, transport and flowers

Table 9.14 continued

Ages	Manifestations	Stages
6½ yr	Reception	Completely competent for all home, school and neighbourhood situations
	Expression	Spoken language fully intelligible, grammatical and fluent. Engages in elaborate make-believe play and win/lose team games with chosen friends, explaining rules and objectives lucidly. Draws more elaborate 'pictures' showing people and objects in all sorts of everyday situations. Interested in learning to read, write and calculate

Play

'Play' defies definition. Sheridan (1975b) suggested that it was an eager participation in physical and/or mental effort with emotional satisfaction. Brunner (1974) stressed that what characterized play was the approach to it rather than the actual content.

To say that something is playful is to suggest that it is not serious, yet the play of a young child can be very intense and appear to be very serious.

Many of the waking hours of a young child are spent in play, so we need to understand what constitutes play at this age (Matterson, 1965; Tizard and Harvey, 1977; Smith and Evans, 1985).

Practice play

As each new skill and understanding is acquired, children have an urge to practise it, and such activity comes to dominate their behaviour for a period of time which can vary from a few days to months. An early example is 'casting', when a child has realized that objects have an existence both in their hands and also on the surrounding floor. A later example is preoccupation with being a cowboy by a boy who has recently reached an understanding of role play.

Observation of practice play shows the most recent level reached by the child. Prolonged persistence of practice play should cause concern and lead to an investigation of the cause.

Exploratory play

Play can be a great voyage of discovery. In the earlier years, exploration forms a large part of play. Observation of a young child requires not only a note of what they can do, but also the uses to which they put their abilities.

An aspect of exploratory play consists of pulling things apart to find out what they are made of and what makes them work. Such play in moderation is understandable, but in excess can be destructive and needs to be inhibited.

Imaginative play (Singer, 1973)

A number of features are included under this title, including symbolization, transference of identity, and role play.

Symbolization, as described elsewhere, is the understanding that items can be represented in various ways, such as by models, drawings and names. A child's play shows his level of symbolic understanding, and the play provides the opportunity to reinforce and advance this understanding.

An extension of symbolization is seen in children's ability to transfer identities to all manner of objects. Thus a large box can be turned over to represent a bus one day and a boat another. This pretend play can become quite complex. It occurs at a stage of early social interaction, so often three or four children are involved.

Not only can children transfer identities to objects around themselves, but they can assume new identities themselves. The identities they take on are usually familiar figures in their everyday life, or striking characters from television scenes or books. In role play, children often act out the activities they see around them, such as becoming the milkman and delivering the milk and taking orders for the next day. At this stage, observing a group of children at play can be as entertaining as a visit to the theatre.

Social play

Early play involves the baby and mother. When mobility develops there is opportunity for play away from mother and solitary play becomes more frequent. Circumstances may tend to inhibit solitary play, as in large families and on occasions when children are put together in nurseries. For those children who seem to be always surrounded by others, it is important to create opportunities for solitary play. For those children who are always on their own, a surfeit of solitary play can be detrimental.

When young children play together, much time may be spent on preserving their possessions, and squabbles arise when one takes a car or doll or bucket from another child. They come to appreciate and tolerate play together, but it is *parallel play*, with each doing his own thing.

An ability to share, an understanding of taking turns and the performance of a joint co-operative activity are all later developments. By this time, children are becoming ready for the regimentation and discipline of school life.

Language and play

Play may be silent, but even then inner language may have an essential role in its organization and progress. On other occasions the verbalizations accompanying play merit attention. They may be directing the play or interpreting it. They reveal much about a child's understanding and thinking. Play provides a good medium for the use and practice of language skills (Le Normand, 1986).

Emotions and play

The pattern of a child's play often reflects his emotional state, and observation can provide insights into his fears, anxieties, love and tenderness. Children under stress may use play as an outlet to express and resolve their problems. Structured play activities are used in child psychiatric practice.

Learning and play

Through play children learn – to know and understand the world around them, how much they can do, how to relate with others, and something about themselves. The potential learning opportunities of play are immense, but debate rages about how much children learn from free play and how much play has to be structured and organized. Free play provides full scope for the child's spontaneity, avoids adult dominance, and encourages independence and self-reliance. Organized play is probably more efficient in ensuring that certain topics are learnt.

Adults and play

Mothers are the first adults in any child's life. Although differing widely from their babies in size and abilities, mothers interact with them as one unit. Some mothers continue this relationship as their babies grow and become their first playmates. Others, however, adopt a more supervisory and directing adult role.

In the early years, adults can decide how they play with children – whether at the child's level or at a more detached level. Children show by their response which they prefer and are used to.

Older children like to play with adults and feel they are growing up.

Development of attention

Babies' early reactions occur in response to internal stimuli such as hunger, but all their senses are assailed by many external stimuli which in time come to have more influence. In order to progress they have to learn to recognize and to deal with these external stimuli, but there are too many of them so they have to acquire ability to give attention selectively. Babies who fail to develop such inhibitory powers become confused and irritable.

Study of the development of attention in the early years provides insights into cognitive development, and clues to the successful conduct of examinations. The changes are summarized in Table 9.15.

Table 9.15 Development of attention

Approximate age period	Characteristics	Significance
First 6 mth	Internal stimuli have strong effect. Awareness of multiple stimuli from a small area around them. A strong external stimulus within their small area of interest will get their attention but responses may be slow	Make allowance for state of baby in examination (see Table 6.2). Allow time for responses
Second 6 mth	Internal stimuli less strong. Switch attention to new strong external stimulus increasingly promptly	Ideal period for distraction tests
1–1½ yr	More selective in response to external stimuli and may ignore if uninteresting or repetitive. Once given, attention may be sustained	Examiner needs to be skilful – introducing new stimulus when attention wanes. Timing is important
1½–2½ yr	Attention once given is single channelled and may be absolute, with rejection of other stimuli. Behaviour rigid and negative	Patience and tact needed. Avoid confrontation. Tantrums may occur
2½–3½ yr	Attention still single channelled, but intensity decreasing. Beginning to gain own control of switching	Adults more successful in switching attention, especially when using encouragement
3½–5 yr	Has become able to switch attention from one stimulus to another in sequence. Later able to give attention to simultaneous stimuli	Now responsive to interchange in play, and to direction

Cognitive development (Isaacs, 1966; Newsom and Newsom, 1970; Mussen, Conger and Kagen, 1974)

Cognitive development during the first five years is very considerable indeed, as is apparent by watching what children do and listening to what they say. Many aspects are covered in the descriptions of play and language and other abilities above.

Initially they are avid for knowledge – 'what's this?', 'why that?'. Later they recognize differences and similarities and begin to group and classify items. They understand the purpose of many items and will act out actions either themselves or in their play. An ability to transfer identity appears to assist their learning. Thus, a box can be a bus as they learn to understand about travel activities in their play, and a doll will become a person as they learn about relationships.

Towards the end of the period there is more evidence of abstract thinking and of reasoning – 'what will happen if?'.

The advances which occur between 3 and 5 years were shown when two children were asked about dressing. When a 3 year old was asked if she could put on her coat, she got her coat and put it on. The thought and the action were linked at this age. When a 5 year old was asked the same question, she said 'yes of course' – at 5 she was able to deal with the situation in a detached way.

Emotional development (Isaacs, 1964; Brackbill and Thompson, 1967)

This is a tumultuous period, during which extremes of behaviour occur and problems frequently concern distraught parents. The era of the 'terrible twos' and 'traumatic threes' is well named.

Behaviour is the response to several influences and an important one is the child's own feelings. It is wrong, however, to attribute all behaviour to the child; to think that a child's feelings are always shown in his behaviour; and that a child with 'bad' behaviour has 'bad' feelings.

At the end of the first year a child's recently acquired mobility plunges him into a wider world and creates the prospects of moving away from his parents and achieving independence. The emotional conflict between secure attachment and uncertain detachment rages. He is also learning a lot about his new wide world, and he is beginning to realize he is an independent being who can control his surroundings. Little wonder then that his behaviour may be totally subdued as he feels overwhelmed by these influences, or may be very aggressive as he demonstrates his new-found feeling of independence, or may fluctuate rapidly between the two.

At this stage his feelings tend to be strong and overwhelming. Thus when sad, he is distraught; when happy, he bubbles over with joy. His strong feelings lead to excessive manifestations. Struggles occur between child and parents as the latter try to control and train their child. Discipline never seems right – either too lax and allowing the child to control the situation, or too restrictive and inhibiting all but the most determined and flamboyant of children.

Feelings and reactions occur in the here and now. Awareness of the past and future has not developed, but when it does towards the end of this age period the child becomes more relaxed and conforming.

As the child passes the autocratic phase of 2 and 3 years his feelings modify and mature and his behaviour changes accordingly. Having demonstrated his independence, he can relax now and begin to show love and acceptance of his parents, and begin to play alongside other children.

The active make-believe world of the threes and fours may be accompanied by imaginary fears and fancies. Nightmares are experienced.

A 5 year old wants to please. He feels happy when praised and sad when criticized. He wants to co-operate and help. He is socially mature and ready to join the group at school.

Exhibition of extreme patterns of behaviour

Very wide variations of behaviour are seen during this period. A shy timid child may be just as normal as an uninhibited extrovert. Nevertheless, persistent marked extremes of behaviour, sudden change in the usual pattern of behaviour, and behaviour inappropriate to the circumstances may all indicate abnormality. The very withdrawn child should be easy to spot, but may be overlooked because he has 'no problem'. The uninhibited socializer who goes to anyone yet fails to make any deep and lasting relationships may be seriously abnormal, despite the fact that his parents may think he is very bright. Gaze avoidance is particularly significant of probable abnormality.

References

Arnheim, D. D. and Pestolesi, R. A. (1973) *Developing Motor Behaviour in Children.* St. Louis: C. V. Mosby

Barsley, M. (1966) *The Left-handed Book.* London: Pan Books, Cox and Wyman

Bayley, N. (1965) *Bayley Infant Scales of Development* (revised) *Mental and Motor.* New York: Psychological Corporation

Bender, L. (1938) *A Visual Motor Gestalt Test and Its Clinical Use.* New York: American Orthopsychology Association

Benton, A. L. (1959) *Right–Left Discrimination and Finger Localisation.* New York: Harper & Rowe

Brackbill, Y. and Thompson, G. G. (1967) *Behaviour in Infancy and Early Childhood.* New York: The Free Press

Brunner, J. S. (1974) The nature and use of immaturity. In *The Growth of Competence* (eds. Connolly, K. and Bruner, J. S.). London: Academic Press

Buchler, C. and Hetzer, H. (1935) *Testing Children's Development from Birth to School Age.* London: Allen and Unwin

Cooper, J., Moodley, M. and Reynell, J. (1983) *Helping Language Development.* London: Edward Arnold

Di Leo, J. H. (1967) *Young Children and their Drawings.* London: Constable

Duffy, J. K. and Irwin, J. V. (1951) *Speech and Hearing Hurdles.* Columbus, Ohio: School Service

Frankenberg, W. K., Camp, B. W., van Natta, P. A., Demersseman, J. A. and Voor Lees, S. F. (1971) Reliability and stability of the Denver Developmental Screening Test. *Child Dev., **42**, 1315*

Gesell, A. and Amatruda, C. S. (1947) *Developmental Diagnosis of Normal and Abnormal Child Development.* New York: Harper & Row

Goodenough, F. L. (1926) *Measurement of Intelligence by Drawings.* New York: Brace and World

Griffiths, R. (1954) *The Abilities of Babies.* London: University Press

Harris, D. B. (1963) *Children's Drawings as Measures of Intellectual Maturity.* New York: Brace and World

Holt, K. S. (1965) *The Assessment of Cerebral Palsy.* London: Lloyd Luke

Horton, M. E. and Rosenbloom, L. (1971) The maturation of fine prehension in young children. *Devl. Med. Child Neurol., **13**, 3*

Illingworth, R. S. (1966) *Development of the Infant and Young Child; Normal and Abnormal,* 3rd edn. Edinburgh: Livingstone

Isaacs, S. (1964) *Social Development in Young Children.* London: Routledge and Kegan Paul

Isaacs, S. (1966) *Intellectual Growth in Young Children.* London: Routledge and Kegan Paul

Kay, H. (1970) Analysing motor skill performance. In *Mechanisms of Motor Skill Development* (ed. Connolly, K. H.), p. 139. London: Academic Press

Keogh, J. (1965) *Motor Performance of Elementary School Children.* Berkeley: Department of Physical Education, University of California

Le Normand, M. T. (1986) A developmental exploration of language used to accompany symbolic play in young normal children (2–4 years). *Child Care Hlth Dev., 12,* 121–134

McCaskill, C. L. and Wellman, B. L. (1938) A study of common motor achievements at the pre-school ages. *Child Dev., 9,* 141

Matterson, E. M. (1965) *Play with a Purpose for the Under 7's.* London: Pelican Books

Mussen, P. H., Conger, J. J. and Kagen, J. (1974) *Child Development and Personality,* 4th edn. New York: Harper and Row

Neligan, G. and Prudham, D. (1969) Norms for four standard developmental milestones by sex, social class and place in family. *Devl. Med. Child Neurol., 11,* 423

Newsom, J. and Newsom, E. (1970) *4 Years Old in an Urban Community.* London: Pelican Books

Reynell, J. K. (1969) A developmental approach to language disorders. *Br. J. Disord. Comm., 4,* 33

Rheingold, H. L. (1960) The measurement of maternal care. *Child Dev., 31,* 565

Sheridan, M. D. (1960) *The Developmental Progress of Infants and Young Children.* London: HMSO

Sheridan, M. D. (1969) Vision screening procedures for very young or handicapped children. *Clinics Dev. Med. 32.* London: Heinemann

Sheridan, M. D. (1975a) The Stycar language test. *Devl. Med. Child Neurol., 17,* 164

Sheridan, M. D. (1975b) The importance of spontaneous play in the fundamental learning of handicapped children. *Child Care Hlth Dev., 1,* 3–17

Singer, J. L. (ed.) (1973) *The Child's World of Makebelieve.* New York: Academic Press

Slosson, H. (1963) *Intelligence Test for Children and Adults.* New York: Slosson Education Publications

Smith, P. K. and Evans, R. (1985) Children's play. *Early Child Dev. Care,* special edn., *19,* 1–132

Stutsman, R. (1948) *Mental Measurement of Preschool Children.* New York: Harcourt and World

Terman, L. M. and Merrill, M. A. (1937) *Measuring Intelligence.* Boston: Houghton Mifflin

Tizard, B. and Harvey, D. (1977) Biology of play. *Clinics Dev. Med. 62.* London: Heinemann

Touwen, B. C. L. (1972) Laterality and dominance. *Devl. Med. Child Neurol., 14,* 747

Valentine, C. W. (1985) *Intelligence Tests for Children,* 6th edn. London: Methuen

Chapter 10

Developmental characteristics and examination at certain ages from 1 to 5 years

Review of development in the first five years

18 months old

The 18 month olds should be walking. Many have been doing so for a few months and are now effective toddlers, seldom falling, able to bend in order to pick up an object from the floor, to modify the speed of walking, and to carry a plaything as they move about. They play with large push and pull toys. They explore and play with almost anything, but seem particularly to enjoy everyday household objects with which they demonstrate their understanding of purpose by imitating domestic activities.

Awareness of different parts of the body is just developing and they show this by pointing to their shoes and taking off their hats and socks.

At 18 months manipulative skills are developing rapidly as shown by their successful use of a spoon in feeding, which they do without tipping it over and spilling. They are also able to build a small tower of two or three cubes, and given a crayon they will scribble on paper.

Their language is developing and most will have a few words which they use correctly, and which are usually the names of everyday objects. They enjoy pointing out familiar items in pictures. Their vocalizations, however, are seldom limited to just a few words. Long babbled conversations – jargon – are heard frequently, and singing may be attempted. Simple games of 'peekaboo' and 'give and take' are enjoyed and may lead to peals of laughter. They carry out simple single instructions, e.g. 'Bring Mummy's handbag'.

Examination at 18 months

Enquiry:	Any problems? – especially with regard to feeding, sleeping, behaviour.
Observation:	Of method of moving about, e.g. walking, running, pushing large-wheeled toy and uses made of these abilities. Spontaneous play with cubes, cup and spoon, small hair brush, doll. Note also any vocalizations, especially number of words, phrases, intonation, clarity and meaning.
Measurement:	(best at end of examination), weight, head circumference.
Examination:	Ears – auroscopy and tympanometry if indicated. A free field hearing test can be performed using the objects available for play. The child sits on the mother's knee in front of a table on which the

objects are set out – ideally five items, but three or four if the child is confused by more. The child is asked with a very quiet spoken voice (not whisper) to point to one of the items. The examiner can also use his own voice to produce high-frequency sounds.

Eyes – near vision. Ability to detect 'hundreds and thousands' (as described earlier). Sonksen picture cards (Sonksen and Macrae, 1987); other examinations if indicated.

Cover test for latent strabismus and mounted balls test (Chapter 8). It should be possible to perform the latter test at 6 m and to examine each eye separately. In addition, convergence and following are checked and ophthalmoscopy performed if indicated.

Manipulation: The child is encouraged to build a tower with cubes.

General medical and neurological examinations are performed if indicated.

2 years old

Two year olds are extremely energetic. They are able to walk and run, to stop and start with ease, to avoid colliding with objects, and to squat to play with an object and to rise again. They climb onto furniture, crawl upstairs, seat themselves at table, and go wherever they can contrive to reach. Doors and drawers may not be barriers. They are just beginning to attempt to throw and to kick. They still tend to misjudge sizes and distances, e.g. they may try to sit in a doll's chair, or walk into a ball when trying to kick it. But these mistakes are being corrected. Considerable variations are seen between children, depending to some extent on their experiences.

Language has greatly developed in the preceding 6 months. They now understand many words and will use 50 or more different words, many of which are articulated clearly. They will put two or three words together. They ask for things by name. *Jargon* is disappearing, and *echolalia* is appearing. They like to listen to stories and to join in songs and nursery rhymes.

They will hold a book and turn the pages one by one. They understand requests and enjoy doing little errands.

They have a strong sense of their own identity and possessions. They resist anything being done to them, e.g. medical examinations, and they safeguard their possessions and will often have a tantrum if a favourite one is taken away.

Many children of this age are feeding themselves and some are clean and dry, but others may still be having intense battles over one or other of these items.

In play, domestic mimicry is very evident; so also is an interest in simple building and screwing tasks. They are beginning to understand that an object can be represented by its name (verbal labelling) and by a model, picture or drawing (symbolization). This new appreciation of the identity and representation of objects may result in their distress if they see them incomplete or broken and they will attempt to make them whole again. Preferred hand use is usually evident. They will hold a pencil like a rod and scribble on paper. They build up cubes and usually succeed in making a tower of six or seven cubes before it falls.

Examination at 2 years
Similar to 18 months. Especial attention should be given to pattern of play and verbalizations.

3 years old

Children are not miniature adults, but anyone meeting a 3-year-old child for the first time might be forgiven for thinking he was. The 3 year old is no longer a toddler. Boys play with tools, cars and engines, but girls are often seen talking to their dolls. It is interesting to speculate how much their greater opportunity for playing with dolls contributes to girls' superiority in language development as compared with boys at this age. They hold conversations with both adults and their playthings. They identify themselves with adults, especially their mothers, with whom they are affectionate and confiding. Their engagement in domestic tasks is no longer simple imitation, but acting out their mothers' roles. This role adoption is extended further and is shown in the vivid make-believe play which appears at this age and which they may share with playmates and siblings.

Very often, observation of play reveals a child's expressive language development. Speech is well developed, is supported by an extensive vocabulary, and is fairly clear apart from some persisting infantile phonetic patterns. He tells his name and sex, asks questions, recites nursery rhymes, and converses about many things including absent objects and past experiences.

Language is used to direct and to control play. So rich is language development at this stage and so valuable for play and intellectual development, that it seems amazing that some children who do not develop speech and language until quite late do not suffer more general effects and frustration than they appear to do.

Counting, and a sense of quantity, are just beginning to appear, as is also an understanding of sharing and taking turns.

The 3 year old is independent with regard to some aspects of undressing, dressing and washing, but still needs some assistance and supervision.

He is nimble on his feet, and is fairly accurate in judging positions and sizes of openings. Motor skills are now well established and proficient. He negotiates steps, going up with alternating feet, but going down he may still put two feet on each step. He likes to jump, and can stand on one leg momentarily. He is now beginning to ride a tricycle and to throw and catch a ball, albeit very immaturely.

Manipulative skills include building a tower of eight or nine cubes; holding a pencil in a conventional way and copying a circle; cutting with scissors; threading beads.

Examination at 3 years

Enquiry:	Any problems? – especially of play and activities, speech, relationships. Experience of playgroup or nursery.
Observation:	Movements in walking and running. Provide a large and a small ball and note kick, catch and throw. Allow spontaneous play with cubes, doll's tea-set, pencil and paper.
Measurement:	Weight, possibly also height, head circumference, blood pressure.
Examination:	Ears: auroscopy and tympanometry if indicated.
	Hearing: identification of suitable pictures to quietly spoken voice (e.g. Michael Reed pictures), repetition of spoken words and phrases.

Eyes: convergence and following. Cover test (see Chapter 8.)

Vision: near vision – 'hundreds and thousands' (see Chapter 8). Vision at 6 m each eye. Separately – mounted balls test (see Chapter 8).

Manipulation: use cubes to make train with chimney and three-cube pyramid. Use pencil and paper to reproduce a stroke, circle and cross.

Language: present picture cards of everyday activities (e.g. Ladybird Books) and note ability to name and describe actions.

Bus Puzzle test (Egan and Brown, 1984a). In this test the child is presented with an attractive board showing a street scene with a bus as a dominant feature. Various items are removable as with a formboard. It is easy to use because children are interested in it. It tests ability to remove and replace the parts and a range of language functions, from naming to answering questions about the different items. It is designed to cover the age range from 20 to 48 months and is especially appropriate at 3 years.

When necessary, a general medical and neurological examination can be performed.

4 years old

Four-year-old children walk and run skilfully, turning and negotiating objects at speed. Stairs no longer present problems; they go up them easily with alternating feet without needing support, and in most cases are as nimble going down. They climb whenever they get a chance. Many are now able to balance on one leg for a few seconds, and this leads to hopping. Those who have had the opportunity to practise may now be expert tricycle riders.

A 4 year old should be able to eat well with a spoon and to use a knife when required. Knowing the front and back of clothes, he should be able to undress and dress completely, except for buttons, back fastenings and laces. He should wash and dry his face and hands and brush his teeth.

Four year olds are aware of their own toilet needs and most will attend to these themselves. Boys will stand to urinate in imitation of their fathers. Both boys and girls should be able to sit on a normal size toilet seat, but they may still need to be checked and helped with wiping themselves.

Their grip upon a pencil is now almost at the mature dynamic tripod stage, with the thumb and first two fingers flexibly controlling the pencil point as they copy a circle and a cross and attempt to draw a house and a man.

They can exhibit skill and understanding in numerous ways: with cubes, by building a bridge from a model, and a three-cube pyramid; with pencil and paper, by copying a circle and a cross, and by folding a piece of paper twice or three times; with formboards, by completing them within a specified time; and with various objects, by selecting them according to differences in size, weight, length and colour.

A four year old's speech is now free of most of the earlier infantile phonetic substitutions. He is constantly questioning, and also recounting his own experiences. He is apt to exaggerate and enjoys fantasy stories, incongruities and jokes.

In social activities he likes companionship both with other children and with adults. He has bouts of quarrelsomeness as well as close co-operation. He appears to have some feeling for others. Now that he has an understanding of time, he looks forward to treats and trips.

5 years old

Almost all 5-year-old children enjoy exhibiting their motor skills – hopping, skipping with alternate feet, dancing rhythmically to music, sliding, swinging and playing ball games with sufficient ability to begin to join in group games. These characteristics are utilized at children's parties and ballet lessons.

Manipulative skills have advanced and are put to many uses. A 5 year old will hold a pencil maturely and enjoy drawing and painting. He draws a recognizable person and house. The figures he draws have limbs and facial features, and his houses have doors and windows. He now copies a triangle and a square. Some 5 year olds are even able to write a few letters.

He should be almost, if not completely, independent in everyday skills such as dressing, washing and eating. He goes on simple errands and will help his mother in the house.

In play he enjoys dressing up and make-believe. He shows understanding of the needs of others and plays companionably with other children. He picks his friends. He both understands something about rules and also finds them acceptable.

His language shows evidence of his understanding. His speech is fluent and grammatically correct. He asks the meaning of abstract words, distinguishes parts of the day, counts to 20 or more, carries out complex commands which require three or four actions, names coins and colours, and appreciates similarities and differences.

Examination at 4 and 5 years

Enquiry:	Any problems? – activities, speech, toilet control, independence, fears and anxieties, friendships.
Observation:	Of composure and responses. Experience of nursery activities, play with pencil and paper, books, cubes, scissors, dolls.
Measurement:	Height and weight.
Examination:	Ears: auroscopy; tympanometry if indicated.

Hearing: Formal audiometry should be possible.

Eyes: movements and convergence. Cover test.

Vision: each eye should be examined separately at 6 m and nearby. Snellen-type letters can now be used (Egan and Brown, 1984b) and suitable ones are the Sheridan–Gardiner and the Sonksen–Silver tests (Sheridan and Gardiner, 1970; Sonksen and Silver, 1988).

Manipulation: with cubes, build six-cube pyramid, bridge and gate. With pencil and paper, reproduce square; Goodenough Draw-a-Man test. Also, bead threading, pegboard, and use of scissors.

Language: engage in conversation using pictures as prompt. Nursery rhymes.

At this age, a general medical and neurological examination are useful.

Signs of abnormality: 1–5 years

These are years of very rapid development. Many new skills appear, and each day presents numerous opportunities (or should do) to practise and to elaborate upon them. Lateness of development, clumsy, inept and bizarre performance of actions, and failure to utilize opportunities may all indicate abnormality. Parents seek help when their child is noticeably slower than his contemporaries, and especially if he is not walking or talking when other children are doing so. They may also seek help if their child's actions and behaviour seem to be different from other children, or from what they expect, and also if they find difficulty in understanding and relating to their child. All these worries must be taken seriously and appraised according to the history and circumstances and the results of examinations.

However, not all delayed and deviant development is due to serious abnormality. With such rapid advances occurring in many aspects of development, considerable individual variations can be expected and do in fact occur. During this period, perhaps more than in any other, is seen the influence of environmental factors and opportunities upon the richness of development. Before deciding that any particular aspect of development is abnormal, the possibility that it may be due to normal variations or to reduced or unused opportunities must be considered.

Developmental delay should be suspected in the following circumstances.

Existence of measurable delay
A quantitative measure of developmental delay in this age range can be obtained from a variety of tests such as the Bayley, Gesell, Griffiths and Merrill–Palmer tests (see Chapter 14). The Reynell Language Scales are particularly useful because they explore several aspects of language development, which is such a prominent and important feature of this period .

Detection of changes in quality of performance
Observation must be made of how a child performs a task, as it often reveals abnormality. Uncertainty, clumsiness, tremor, posturing of the hands and poor eye–hand co-ordination may be noticed.

Persistence of earlier patterns
Abnormality should be suspected when some earlier aspect of behaviour persists longer than should be the case. Some activities not only persist too long, but are exaggerated and dominate the child's behaviour.

Casting, for example, is normally seen at the beginning of the second year and does not normally persist more than a month or two. Casting is the name given to the activity in which the child delights in dropping his toys off the tray of his high-chair or out of his pram. It is as if he were practising his newly acquired awareness of the continuity of objects in space and time as he throws them from one place to another. Normally, during the few months casting is present it can be used by an understanding mother as a game. Each time she picks up the toys she talks, laughs and tickles her baby. In this way the opportunities for reinforced interpersonal relationships which it provides are fully utilized. However, persistence of casting beyond 18 months, its exaggeration and the failure of the child to develop more fruitful activities indicate probable abnormality. Similarly, a certain amount of echolalia is normally heard around 2–2½ years, but its persistence should make the doctor very suspicious of abnormality.

References

Egan, D. F. and Brown, R. (1984a) Developmental assessment. Eighteen months to four-and-a-half years. The Bus Puzzle test. *Child Care Hlth Dev.*, **10**, 381–390

Egan, D. F. and Brown, R. (1984b) Vision testing of young children in the age range 18 months to 4½ years. *Child Care Hlth. Dev.*, **10**, 381–390

Sheridan, M. D. and Gardiner, P. A. (1970) Sheridan–Gardiner test for visual acuity. *Br. Med. J.*, **2**, 102–109

Sonksen, P. M. and Macrae, A. J. (1987) Vision for coloured pictures at different acuities: the Sonksen picture guide to visual function. *Devl. Med. Child Neurol.*, **29**, 337–347

Sonksen, P. M. and Silver, J. (1988) *The Sonksen–Silver Acuity System*. Windsor: Keeler Ltd.

Chapter 11

Development in the school years

Development of the younger school child: 6–10 years

These are years of steady progress. They are 'the benign years' because they come between the fervour of rapid development in the first five years and the turbulence of adolescence.

At the beginning of this period the child possesses many motor and language skills, and a considerable degree of independence both in self-care activities and sense of personal identity. He is ready for systematic training to perfect his skills and to use them to increase his knowledge and understanding, and it is customary to arrange his training in similar age groups. Entry into this new world of peer groups within school, and adjustment to the situation, is a characteristic feature of the beginning of this period.

Physical growth proceeds at a steady rate during these years, with almost identical increments of height and weight each year. Strength increases. Sex differences are present: boys are bigger and stronger than girls and succeed better in motor skills requiring strength, whereas girls tend to be lighter and more nimble.

Motor skills are developed for useful activities, such as running, jumping, climbing, swimming, riding. Both unorganized frolics, such as tree climbing, and organized games promote the steady evolution of motor abilities. So many activities can be developed that it is not always possible to have the time to become skilful in all of them. Even so, some junior school children do remarkably well in this respect. A good foundation of motor skills in the early years is a help to them, and they are also urged on by the natural competitiveness of this period and a desire to gain approval from their peers. Personal interests and opportunities determine which skills are favoured and there is a strong culturally determined sex difference; for example, girls skip and knit and boys climb and do woodwork.

A great ability to absorb information both aurally and visually develops in this period. No opportunity is lost by school teachers and sometimes parents to pour knowledge into the receptive youngsters. Evidence of these pressures may be seen sometimes in the children's performance and reactions. For example, it seems possible that the recent trend to focus attention less on what a child says and how he speaks and more on his ability to read has led to a decline in problems of stuttering and an increase in reading disabilities.

One of the most important developments in this period is an increase of conceptual ability. There are increases in concept formation, the complexity of the conceptualization, and the ability to formulate hypotheses. These all arise from the language development of earlier years. To form concepts the child has to have ability to categorize and group his impressions. Then he is able to begin to understand their meaning, purpose and interrelationships. He develops concepts of quantity (mass), number, distance and spatial relationships; of values in money; and of more abstract ideas of good and bad and beautiful and ugly. He comes to have ideas about life and death, and of past, present and future. As with all emerging abilities, he likes to practise his mastery of concepts whenever he can. He enjoys fantasies in which real and unreal situations merge; is fascinated by extremes such as the grotesquely huge and minutely small; and is intrigued by riddles which introduce possible misconceptions. His concepts of good and bad often create a fear of being bad and of being disapproved of by his parents, or by a more remote parent figure of God.

Conceptualization helps him to learn about and to understand his world and himself. To match this broader comprehension, his world expands as he enters school and he is more active outside the home. He achieves greater emancipation from adult support and direction, and develops identification with and reliance upon peer groups.

Children who fail to gain acceptance by a peer group lose more than the widening of experiences which comes from such association. They carry their own thoughts and feelings, may feel sad and lonely, and may brood.

At the end of this period the child has gained physical, intellectual, emotional and social strengths. His understanding of the world and his abilities make him a pleasant companion for adults, and even encourage moments of cheekiness. Carried to extremes these features create the aggressive single-sex groups of this age. Puberty is not far off, however, when many changes will take place.

The overwhelming characteristic of this period appears to be a striving towards certain goals – physical, intellectual and emotional. Many things enhance, inhibit or distort these changes and in consequence great variations are seen between children of similar ages. Clear-cut developmental levels are not as evident as in the earlier years. Any individual child should be judged by the relative strength of these developmental features. For example, peer-group identification develops during this age period. In any particular child this characteristic may, or may not, be well marked and may occur early or late during this period, but usually peer-group identification is shown only weakly by most 7-year-old children and much more strongly with 9 year olds.

A summary of the developmental features of the period from 5 to 10 years is shown in Table 11.1.

Development of motor skills

Between 6 and 10 years of age many motor skills develop and improve. Strength, speed, accuracy and neatness all improve and reflect the considerable amount of motor learning which takes place. Figure 11.1 shows the increasing proficiency of some motor skills during this age period (Keogh, 1965).

Development of writing

This skill requires that the child steady the paper with one hand while holding the writing implement in an appropriate way with the other. He must recognize the nature of the task and then reproduce the letter symbols on the paper. At first the

Table 11.1 Overview of development, 5–10 years

Age (yr)	Area of activity	Motor abilities	Manipulation	Daily activities	Personal–social	Language
5	Home Infant school	Stands on one leg Hops Jumps off step	Draws with dynamic tripod	Goes simple errands	Parents and adults held in awe; active imagination, fears and fantasies, exaggerations, tells tales	Increasing ability to express thoughts and use language directively
6				Manages own daily care, e.g. dressing, going to bed	Increasing link to peer group, but still needs adult support and direction	New concepts developing rapidly; greater understanding of size, shape, weight, distance, etc.
7	Junior school	Runs, climbs	Prints, large irregular letters	May get self to school	Ideals of right; God as punitive super-father	
8					Needs acceptance by peers; resents social isolation	Ability to hypothesize and solve problems beyond the here and now
9–10	Increasing activity outdoors, parks, etc.	All skills performed more smoothly and efficiently; competitive games	Joined up, neat writing; bat and ball games	Beginning to help in household tasks, e.g. washing up, making tea. Increasing reliability when doing tasks	Tendency to brood; single-sex gangs	

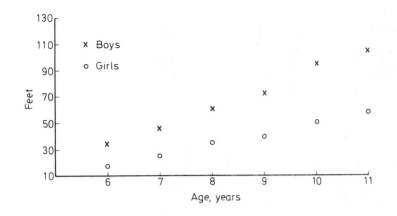

(a)

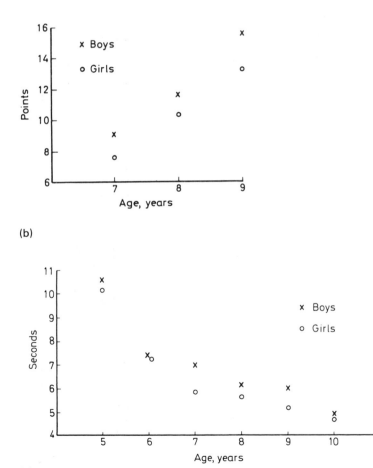

(b)

(c)

Figure 11.1 Some motor skills of school children: (a) ball throw; (b) accuracy of throw; (c) 50 ft (15 m) hop

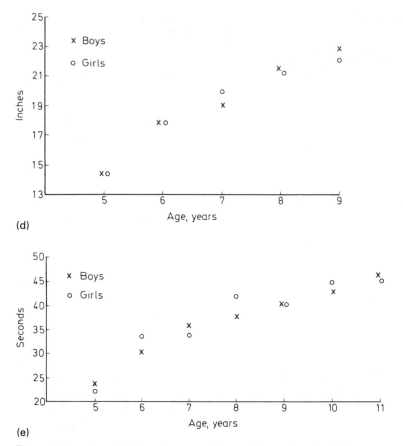

(d)

(e)

Figure 11.1 continued: (d) hurdle jump; (e) beam balance (Keogh, 1965)

letters are poorly formed, of varying sizes and arranged irregularly. These features gradually improve until mature, neat, legible joined-up writing emerges.

Writing is a means of expression, so that what is written is more important than how it is written. Nowadays, encouragement of expression takes precedence over drilling in penmanship. Nevertheless, it is not possible completely to separate these two aspects. Some children experience considerable frustration because they cannot write as quickly as they think and in these cases helping them to achieve an easier, simpler and quicker technique of writing is of value.

With so many factors involved in the development of writing, it is to be expected that wide variations will be encountered. The pattern of evolution of writing skills shown in Figure 11.2 should, therefore, be used only as a general guide and in no way at all as a test.

Development of reading (Schonell and Goodacre, 1974)

Reading is another complex ability acquired during the school years. It requires an ability to recognize letters and words and to understand the meaning of groups of words in sentences. Evidence of such ability is shown by the child responding to a

Age	Characteristics of writing	Example
Up to 5 years	Enjoys using pencil to make patterns. Prints large irregular capitals anywhere on the page. Copies printed words.	*We went to / We we h+ +o / the shops. / +h θ sh o p s*
5–6 years	Prints first name. Letters large and irregular and frequently reversed. Makes erratic attempts at short messages.	*I went to / Church on Sunday / I Sang Songs*
6–7 years	Prints alphabet and numbers 1–20. Copies words. Letters usually capitals. Still large and irregular and sometimes reversed.	*I liked the firewk / they wru very / pittre and I like / the fire to*
7–8 years	Most children can now write and many are struggling to make smaller letters and to set out the writing more neatly. Errors still occur.	*i like rugger because / I like getting durty bu I / have nevr played whth a / propr rugger ball because I havet / got a propr ball.*
8–9 years	Some children are beginning to join letters together. There is often variation in neatness and legibility. Girls tend to be more capable than boys.	*Autumn is passing / winter is coming / Leaves are falling / to the ground*
9–11 years	Writing should be well established and evidence of a joined-up style should be emerging.	*Colder, colder every day / Untill the snow comes / falling falling from the sky.*
11–14 years	Gradual emergence of a fast, legible style of handwriting.	*Bonfire night is when you enjoy yourself. Fire winds in flames in the air from the bright bonfire. Fireworks bang and pop.*

Figure 11.2 Evolution of writing skills (Hurlock, 1956; Jarman, 1973, by permission)

written message, by carrying out a request contained in the message, by laughing at the humour of the written sentences, or by some other appropriate way. The ability to repeat the written sentence verbally, as in reading aloud, is an important attribute and is practised while learning to read. Reading aloud should be associated with comprehension, otherwise the so-called reading is nothing more than mechanical repetition. Unfortunately, forceful emphasis upon learning to read in a narrow sense may produce this type of mechanical reading without comprehension, and should be avoided.

Very many factors contribute to the development of reading ability, so there are wide variations in children's abilities. Reading ability is affected also by the different reading methods which are in use and the opportunities and encouragement received by each child. It is difficult, therefore, to quote precise standards for reading.

There are three major phases which merge into each other. These are as follows:

(a) pre-reading phase – up to 6 years or thereabouts;
(b) reading practice – from about 6 to 9 years;
(c) use of reading – from about 9 years onwards.

In the pre-reading phase, interest in stories and books is encouraged. Participation in word games both at home and in school promotes further interest and encourages recognition of simple words. For example, the teacher talks about the day's weather and asks the child to identify the appropriate words as she mentions the sun and the rain.

Once the basic skills of reading are achieved, considerable practice is required to enable reading to develop to the point at which it can be used by the child for his own purposes. A series of graded readers are used to provide this practice. The sentences are simple and short and there is much repetition of words and phrases. Large print, attractive illustrations and other means are used to increase interest and simplify the task. As the child gets older these adjuvants are lessened.

The attainment of adequate proficiency in reading enables the child to use this ability for his own purposes – understanding written directions, communicating among friends, learning all that is in the books, and also enjoying the stories. At this stage children are expected to use textbooks for classroom work, and some read for pleasure. A wide range of books are available for pleasure reading which can often be introduced to children through their interests and hobbies, e.g. football, riding and stamp collecting.

The evaluation of reading is a complex task which is best carried out by competent educationalists and psychologists. Children with reading problems are frequently referred to developmental paediatricians either to find out if there are any visual, neurological, developmental, emotional or other causes for the reading problem, or to decide the significance of associated phenomena such as clumsiness.

One of the most usual ways to test a child's reading ability consists of presenting a list of words of increasing complexity and finding how many he can read aloud (comprehension of the meaning of the word is not required in most such tests). Figure 11.3 shows one of the most frequently used reading tests – the Schonell Graded Word reading test (McCulloch, 1965). This test has to be administered and scored in the prescribed way. As an approximation, however, each two lines of 10 words represent about 1 year's advance in reading ability between 6 and 15 years of age.

tree	little	milk	egg	book
school	sit	frog	playing	bun

flower	road	clock	train	light
picture	think	summer	people	something

dream	downstairs	biscuit	shepherd	thirsty
crowd	sandwich	beginning	postage	island

saucer	angel	ceiling	appeared	gnome
canary	attractive	imagine	nephew	gradually

smoulder	applaud	disposal	nourished	diseased
university	orchestra	knowledge	audience	situated

physics	campaign	choir	intercede	fascinate
forfeit	siege	recent	plausible	prophecy

colonel	soloist	systematic	slovenly	classification
genuine	institution	pivot	conscience	heroic

pneumonia	preliminary	antique	susceptible	enigma
oblivion	scintillate	satirical	sabre	beguile

terrestrial	belligerent	adamant	sepulchre	statistics
miscellaneous	procrastinate	tyrannical	evangelical	grotesque

ineradicable	judicature	preferential	homonym	fictitious
rescind	metamorphosis	somnambulist	bibliography	idiosyncrasy

Figure 11.3 Schonell Graded Word reading test

Characteristics at 7 and 9 years

7 years old (Figure 11.4)

Seven-year-old children are typically active, happy and biddable. They find a lot to interest them and a lot to do. They still respond to each idea by doing it rather than by thinking about it, so they seem to be hustling about all the time. Play and chatter absorb them until they sag from fatigue, but a sound sleep restores them and they are off again. They eagerly respond to doing things for parents and teachers whom they regard as all-perfect and all-powerful.

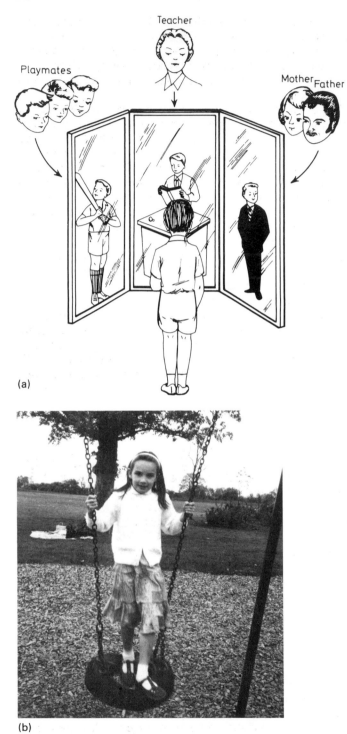

Teacher

Playmates

Mother Father

(a)

(b)

Figure 11.4 Seven years old: (a) development of self-concept; (b) play (Hurlock, 1956)

The years since age 5 have provided the practice for them to become really independent in daily care activities which is accompanied by greatly increased confidence. They defend their rights by fighting, but some of their fights seem really to be no more than a sheer mutual enjoyment of the activity. They boost their own self-esteem by derogatory comments about friends and may still run to tell tales to adults.

Most 7 year olds should be able to read and to write to some extent; the pattern of reading will depend very much upon the type of training they have received. Those trained by the 'look and say' method will read whole words, but may be completely stumped by an unfamiliar word. Those taught by the older phonetic method usually read more slowly as they sound out the syllables, but have more success in sounding out unfamiliar words. Writing usually consists of printing in rather large and irregular letters. Boys especially enjoy physical activity and racing. Climbing and tumbling can develop spontaneously when there are a few together. Football and hand-ball games are played with more efficiency, but some organization by adults may still be necessary.

This is an age when imagination is active; sometimes they will exaggerate their impressions and ideas and quite frighten themselves. Fears of the dark and of frightening films and television can be troublesome.

Their confidence in adults which makes them easy and biddable may also lead to them copying older children. Unless one is careful this can lead them astray.

The 7 year old is at a point of change, with the strength of parental attachments declining and those to the peer groups increasing. Having been with peers for two or so years he is confident in the situation and from now onwards he will increasingly identify with them and hate being different from them in dress, actions and thoughts.

9 years old

The 9-year-old child is growing up and is aware of it. Girls especially are aware that puberty is only a year or two ahead and with it the approach to womanhood. They are beginning to abandon some of their earlier activities as childish. They are less interested in fairy tales. They have a wider interest in everyday affairs and enjoy adventures beyond their everyday world, e.g. trips to museums. An increasing cheekiness is noted, sometimes backed up by reference to friends or 'the gang'.

All motor skills are more assured and quicker than at 7 years. Interest in team games is increasing and is often fostered by interest in a local professional team. Manipulation is good, as shown by neat joined-up handwriting, and by such activities as the making of woodwork articles and the mending of bicycles.

Group identification is very strong. Not only do boys gang together; they positively discourage, deride and reject girls at this stage, and vice versa. Many children of this age are Cubs or Brownies and such activities fulfil their gang interests.

Intellectually the 9 year old is able to deal with many subjects in school, but his powers of understanding abstract relationships are still limited.

Socially, 9-year-old children are still too young to be wholly independent and so they are expected to join in family activities, but they may rebel on occasions. They are capable now of doing more to help and should be encouraged to lay the table, help wash up, clean the car and other suitable activities.

Significance of development: 6–10 years

This is a period of solid learning and steady progress. All skills are practised and are utilized both for learning and reaching independence.

Once the child has settled in school he shows increasing desire and ease of working in peer groups. This is ideal for training the developing minds and greatly facilitates the task of the school teacher.

Everyone recognizes that education does not consist just of pouring in facts, but includes stimulation of the child's interest and exploration and understanding. This is no easy task, and all who desire to help children of this age should understand how they think and learn. Quite often educational failure in this age group is found to be due to an omission or error in some basic concept formation at an earlier stage.

It is all too easy to see the educational aspects of development during these years and to ignore all else. The teacher is teaching and the child is learning. But the child is also learning in the playground and in his home as well as in school, and he is learning about more than is covered by the school curriculum. Not surprisingly, there is ample evidence to show that the more socially advantageous children make better progress than others. The wider aspects of development such as learning to understand himself and his own emotions, and to manage his relationships with others, must be taken into account when evaluating development and behaviour in this period.

Signs of abnormality: 6–10 years

Signs of abnormality usually show themselves in one of three ways: in motor performance, as learning disabilities or as behavioural disturbances.

Clumsiness (Cratty, 1967; Morris and Whiting, 1971)

Clumsiness refers to poor performance in motor skills. Abnormalities of motor performance may be noticed by parents or teachers, and may consist of failure to acquire certain motor skills or their performance in a clumsy or inept fashion. The range of performance encountered normally is extremely wide. Quite poor performance may still be within the normal range, or it might be due to lack of opportunities, or to general illness. These possibilities have to be considered before attributing poor performance to an organic lesion, especially a neurological lesion. The evaluation of the clumsy child is difficult and should always be done by an experienced clinician. Care must be taken, especially by psychologists and teachers, not to speak of brain damage and chronic brain dysfunction without having definite evidence from a specialist medical examination. The evaluation of poor motor performance rests upon a full medical examination, identification of definitely abnormal signs, and above all upon the *quality* of the motor performance and not just what is or is not achieved.

Behind the comment that a child is clumsy may be concern because he is not as good as his fellows, either in what he is able to do or in the speed of his actions; or complaints occur because he is always bumping into things, or dropping things, or is untidy and messy, or has poor handwriting; or anxieties arise because he is not participating with others in games and sports.

In some cases the child is not clumsy at all. His motor skills are perfectly reasonable for his age, but his parents or school may be expecting above-average performances from him. This occurs particularly with the sons of very skilful parents, and with children attending schools where great store is set upon games and athletic prowess.

In other cases the child's inferior performance in motor skills will be confirmed, but this may not be due to pathological causes. There is a very wide range of motor skills in childhood. Some examples are shown in Table 11.2. A 10-year-old girl who can throw a ball only 20 ft (6 m) may seem decidedly feeble, especially as almost all 5-year-old boys will be able to do better, but her performance is well within the 'normal' range for her age and sex. Lack of interest and opportunity may have accentuated her limitations, and she might show improvement with training. Drawing excessive attention to her poor performance and labelling her as clumsy will undoubtedly increase both her difficulties and her reactions to them.

Table 11.2 Wide range of motor skills in childhood: some selected items

Item	Poorest (2 SD)	Average	Best (+2 SD)
5-year-old girls, running 30 yd	6.25 sec	7.67 sec	9.09 sec
5 year olds, hopping 50 ft	31% boys } unable 19% girls } to do it	10.4 sec	
7-year-old boys, grip strength	11.5 lb	26.3 lb	41.1 lb
8 year olds, standing jump	41.6 in	55.2 in	68.8 in
9 year olds, beam balance	16.6 sec	40 sec	63.4 sec
10 year olds, beam walk	15.7 steps	24.3 steps	32.9 steps
10-year-old boys, ball throw	52 ft	94 ft	136 ft
10-year-old girls, ball throw	16.4 ft	49 ft	81.6 ft

The medical management of clumsy children requires considerable skill. Very often an impetuous search for a neurological lesion of 'minimal brain damage' and a desire to apply a diagnostic label is often the most detrimental step possible so far as the child's overall development is concerned. A strategy for the investigation and management of a clumsy child is shown in Table 11.3.

Sometimes, however, a child may be clumsy as a result of a pathological cause. This may be revealed by finding that the motor skills are outside the normal range and that other abnormal features are present. For example, an experienced clinician will notice when excessive movements or unusual postures occur in performing a particular skill and will also be on the look out for grimacing, tremors, ataxia and the presence of mirror movements. The Fog tests are useful in this connection (Fog and Fog, 1963):

Table 11.3 Analysis of child said to be clumsy

Action	Question	Positive response
Child presents as 'clumsy'	Are problems unrelated to motor skills?	E.g. behaviour problems, learning difficulties
Examination	Evidence of neurological disorder?	E.g. ataxia, cerebral palsy
Motor skills test (Stott, Moyes and Henderson, 1972)	Are skills reasonable for chronological?	E.g. high parental expectations
Psychological tests	Are skills reasonable for mental?	Give guidance
Tests of kinesthesis and body awareness (Berges and Lezine, 1965; Laszlo and Bairstow, 1986)	Evidence of defect of motor awareness?	Provide kinesthetic training
Tests of muscle strength and balance	Evidence of defect of motor planning?	Provide therapy
Visual discrimination tests (Frostig *et al.*, 1964)	Evidence of visuo-perceptual problem?	Provide therapy
No positive response to above questions		Advise about strategies to cope and give guidance

1. The child is asked to stand on the lateral borders of his feet with the feet turned inwards. In young children this action causes supination of the arms in most cases, and pronation or extension in others. With increasing age the arm movement is seen less often, and is seldom seen after 10 years of age. The presence of such a reaction above this age is, therefore, an indication of probable abnormality.
2. The child is asked to open a spring clip with the fingers of one hand. In the young there is associated movement of the other hand, but this diminishes with increasing age and is not seen very often after 14 years provided that the clip is not excessively strong. The presence of such a reaction above this age is, therefore, an indication of possible abnormality.

There is no satisfactory test for clumsiness or for motor skill. This statement will not seem surprising after what has been said already about the many factors affecting motor development. Several tests of motor proficiency have been described, notably the Oseretsky, Stott and Gubbay tests (Oseretsky, 1948; Stott, 1966; Gubbay, 1975), which help to identify a clumsy child but do not untangle the various factors involved. Furthermore, these tests include items which are largely dependent upon motor perceptual ability rather than the other components of motor skill and so add to the difficulties of analysing the results.

Rather than trying to solve this situation by tests, the clinical approach recommended is as follows. In the case of a child already labelled as clumsy:

1. Determine if there is impairment of motor skills.
2. Determine the extent of this impairment and the ways it is affecting the child.
3. Determine if there is a pathological cause for the clumsiness. It is important to do this because if it can be shown that there is a definite cause for the

clumsiness, the child cannot be blamed for it. It also helps decide whether training will help or only frustrate, and it gives a guide to future ability. It may further provide some insight into, or forewarning about, associated learning problems.
4. The clumsiness should be analysed to find which components are at fault, e.g. speed, strength, precision, co-ordination and endurance, in order to determine the best ways to overcome the difficulty.

In the case of a child who has not already been labelled as clumsy, but who is found to be so in the course of examination, the above steps should be followed, but caution should be exercised before applying a diagnostic label. On the whole, more harm than help arises from the indiscriminate labelling of children as clumsy.

Learning disabilities
Learning disabilities are more likely to be noticed first by a teacher. In the case of any child who is failing to make educational progress, three areas have to be explored: the child, the content of the teaching, and the teacher and his or her teaching technique. Learning disabilities are far too large a subject to be dealt with here, but it is sufficient to state that all too often these difficulties are not fully investigated, but are dealt with in an *ad hoc* manner.

An example of the factors to be investigated in children with learning difficulties is shown by considering reading impairment.

Learning to read is a complex task. When difficulties arise, search for a cause should be made according to a strategy used for all types of learning difficulty. This strategy consists of asking if the difficulties have arisen as a result of problems with the child, the environment or the subject.

Aspects to be considered with regard to the child:
 Impaired health, now or in the past.
 Sensory impairment, especially visual, and including scanning.
 Intellectual limitation.
 Emotional disturbance.
 Fatigue.
 Low level of interest and motivation.
Aspects to be considered with regard to the environment:
 Uncongenial surroundings.
 Distractions.
 Teaching method – inappropriate, varied and changing.
 Teacher's personality.
Aspects to be considered with regard to the subject:
 Too difficult.
 Too easy.
 Not sufficiently interesting.

Behavioural disorders
Behavioural disorders are extremely difficult to evaluate. Attempts have been made to quantify them, but have not been very satisfactory. The essential point is that any particular behaviour must be seen in the light of the individual child, his past experiences and present circumstances. Two children may behave similarly; the behaviour in one case may be abnormal, yet in the other case the identical behavioural pattern may be normal. The following behavioural features may

indicate abnormality and so call for further attention: extremes of behaviour; change of behaviour; behaviour which is disturbing the child's activities and learning; behaviour which is out of keeping with the child's background and circumstances.

Development of the older school child: 11–15 years

This period of development is concerned with the transition from childhood to adulthood. Hormonal changes produce a considerable spurt in growth at a rate which is often as great as that seen in the second and third years, and they also bring about the appearance of the secondary sexual characteristics. These physical changes in puberty, and a growing awareness of their significance, are associated with emotional changes and reactions which characterize adolescence, especially an increased self-awareness and sexuality.

Motor activities become more organized during this period. There is a peak of interest in team games and competitive events. Personal participation becomes more selective and the choice strongly reflects the child's sex and personality.

Intellectually there is increasing development in complex abstract thought and reasoning. Bright children revel in any intellectual challenge and will join in quiz games and intellectual puzzles. This is just as well because this is a period of intense educational activity in which those with academic prowess are distinguishable (and distinguished) from the others. All too often preoccupation with educational needs leads to neglect of other aspects of development at these ages. It is not surprising that the educational demands of this period are often associated with problems. At present, insufficient attention is given to the medical aspects of these problems, but perhaps this will be remedied in the future.

Although the gang may still have strong appeal at the beginning of this age period, it sooner or later gives way to friendship in smaller groups of two or three. These groups are usually of the same sex, but a desire for heterosexual friendships, either singly or in groups, begins to appear.

The period of gang friendships coincides with rebellion against authority, both parental and also other forms. As the gang period fades, teenagers appear to rebel against parental authority in particular. This often leads to parents considering their children to be thoughtless and difficult, but in fact the children are usually much concerned with ethics and values and are thinking things out. In this process of thinking out they may develop extreme views and intense passions for causes. Religious fervour may occur.

Increasing independence will be seen during this period. Teenagers begin to take responsibility for choosing their own clothes, making their own personal arrangements, and performing more responsible tasks. They respond well to responsibility, for example, when made school prefects. Their increased self-awareness has many repercussions. For example, on the one hand it gives greater insight into the actions and motives of others and, on the other hand, leads to periods of introspection.

Developmental characteristics at 12 and 14 years

12 years old
In Britain this is the first year of the senior school. Puberty comes at different ages and some 12-year-old children will be more physically advanced than others. Quite

wide differences in height are encountered. Differences in physique and interests between boys and girls are becoming even more apparent. Girls are beginning to appear more mature than the boys. There is relatively little mixing between the sexes; both prefer groups of their own sex and usually shun and scorn the other sex. Boys appear to be coarse and clumsy to girls, while girls seem to be silly and giggly to boys. Organized activities, as in Scouts and Guides, are popular and provide a combination of opportunities for adventure which the 12-year-old craves, with the structure and support which he still requires.

Twelve-year-old children tend to be critical of their parents and may even be openly rebellious. This seems to be largely due to a desire to do things for themselves, rather than an appreciation of themselves as adults which becomes more evident later.

14 years old

Most 14-year-old children are well advanced into puberty and, in some, the physical changes will be complete. Both sexes are much nearer to their adult characteristics and in consequence appear to be considerably more mature than 12 year olds. Personal interests and social activities are also more definite and allied to their future adult roles. At this age they like to be treated as emerging young adults and to have opportunities for increasingly independent action and responsibility. These periods last for varying lengths of time and in some 14 year olds may be relatively short and interspersed with periods of return to childishness. This fluctuation between the independence of their adult-like role and the dependence of childhood confuses parents, teachers and, most of all, themselves, in whom it leads to distress and irritation.

The two sexes are quite distinct at this age. Boys are strong and enjoy physical activities. Team games are important, and also opportunities to go adventuring in groups, for example on camping expeditions. Many boys see girls as individuals who cannot attain comparable abilities, and who, when present, disrupt the cohesiveness of the gang. Some regard girls with awe and trepidation, as they sense their future relationships.

Girls at this age are more self-possessed than boys and are more aware of their sexual attractiveness. They often find boys of their own age unattractive because of their lesser maturity. Girls explore the possibilities of self-adornment and will often spend long periods on this activity. This, together with spells of brooding and day-dreaming, makes them seem to be remote from everyday events. In a way they are preparing themselves for a time when they will have to deal with everyday life.

Significance of development and signs of abnormality: 11–15 years

Although the speed of growth and the other physical changes are obvious features of this period, the really significant events are related to the establishment of personalities. Children of this age think about themselves, who they are, why they are, and so forth. They learn much by comparing and contrasting themselves with their parents, their friends, and with idolized figures from the world of entertainment and sport. The processes are not easy and many side effects may be observed. Fluctuations of behaviour, unpredictable reactions and contrariness may all occur frequently during this period. Not surprisingly, educational effort and results may show similar fluctuations.

It is strange that apparently so little attention is given to the developmental needs and stresses during this period which is so often regarded only as an opportunity for more and more teaching. Both physical and emotional adjustments are necessary, and whether the accompanying manifestations are mostly internal or external, severe or mild, they may still be completely normal.

It is particularly difficult to differentiate between normality and abnormality during this period. Gross extremes, both of failure to make the necessary adjustments and of behaviour, should be considered abnormal, if for no other reason than that they require investigation and treatment. Otherwise it is probably far better not to attempt to grade every aspect of behaviour as either normal or abnormal, but to regard it as an expression of the ongoing development.

References

Berges, J. and Lezine, I. (1965) Imitation of gestures. *Clinics Dev. Med. 18.* London: Heinemann

Cratty, B. J. (1967) *Movement Behaviour and Motor Learning,* 2nd edn. London: Kimpton

Fog, E. and Fog, M. (1963) Cerebral inhibition examined by associated movements. *Clinics Dev. Med. 10.* London: Heinemann

Frostig, M., Maslow, P., Lefever, D. W. and Whittlesey, J. R. B. (1964) The Marianne Frostig developmental test of visual perception. *Perceptual and Motor Skills,* **19**, 463–499

Gubbay, S. S. (1975) *The Clumsy Child. A Study of Developmental Apraxia and Agnosic Ataxia.* London: W. B. Saunders

Hurlock, E. (1956) *Child Development,* 4th edn. New York: McGraw-Hill

Jarman, C. (1973) Is children's handwriting neglected? *Where,* 5 Jan.

Keogh, J. (1965) *Motor Performance of Elementary School Children.* Berkeley: Dept of Physical Education, University of California

Laszlo, J. I. and Bairstow, P. (1986) *Perceptual Motor Behaviour.* London: Holt, Rinehart and Winston

McCulloch, R. W. (1965) Review of Schonell tests. In *The Sixth Mental Measurements Year Book* (ed. Buros, O. K.). New Jersey: Gryphon Press

Morris, P. R. and Whiting, H. T. A. (1971) *Motor Impairment and Compensatory Education.* London: Bell and Sons

Oseretsky, N. (1948) Metric scale for studying the motor capacity of children. *J. Consult. Psychol.,* **12**, 37

Schonell, F. J. and Goodacre, E. (1974) *The Psychology and Teaching of Reading,* 5th edn. Edinburgh: Oliver and Boyd

Stott, D. H. (1966) A general test of motor-impairment for children. *Devl. Med. Child Neurol.,* **8**, 523

Stott, D. H., Moyes, F. A. and Henderson, S. E. (1972) *A Test of Motor Impairment.* Windsor: NFER

Part III

Developmental paediatrics

Chapter 12

Developmental diagnosis

A paediatrician's task is to promote the health and development of all children and when abnormalities exist to do all he can to remedy or alleviate them.

Whenever he encounters a child, a paediatrician should be alive to these objectives and should deal with questions raised by parents, teachers, health visitors and anyone else with concern for the child.

The term *surveillance* is applied to tasks of overseeing the health and development of children (Hall, 1988; Butler, 1989).

If problems are suspected, examinations and investigations should be pursued until a clear diagnosis is reached – and this applies to developmental just as much as to health problems.

If the child is considered to be healthy, normal and free of problems, this conclusion must be based upon sound evidence. A quick pronouncement and failure to detect a problem can cause much distress. Errors of this sort have occurred too often in relation to developmental examinations when reliance has been placed on quick 'screening' tests. For example, the free field distraction test for hearing carried out at 7–8 months has a high proportion of false-negative results which actually delays the detection of hearing impairment.

For a period, the *'at risk' concept* was applied to developmental work in the UK. The idea is to identify the precursors of disabling conditions and so define a sub-group of the population with a high risk of abnormalities and then to concentrate attention on this group. The idea did not work well in practice for several reasons:

1. Some precursors of disability could not be defined easily. For example, pre-eclampsia was to be included if severe, but doubts existed about including mild manifestations. Quite often these mild cases were included 'to be on the safe side', and this policy when applied to all factors increased the 'at risk' group beyond manageable proportions.
2. The group not at risk cannot be ignored. It is a low-risk not a no-risk group, and because it contains most of the population just as many problems can come from this group as from the high-risk group.
3. The keeping of 'at risk' registers was sometimes not sufficiently integrated with the day-to-day work in the health clinics.
4. It was shown by Alberman and Goldstein (1970) that only when resources were scarce was it effective to use an 'at risk' group; and when resources were reasonable, attention should be given to the whole population.

There then developed schemes for the examination of all babies and young children at prescribed ages. The term *screening* was applied to this work, but because screening is a well-defined scientific process the term is better avoided or used only for specific items which fulfil the criteria for its satisfactory application.

Screening is the application to a large defined popultion of a simple, safe and reliable test for the early detection of a specific disorder which will respond to treatment.

When considering advocating any screening procedure, attention should be given to the following criteria (Frankenberg, 1974). The proposed test should be *acceptable*:

(a) to the child;
(b) to the parents;
(c) to the teachers;
(d) to others concerned, including religious groups and society;
(e) to those performing the test;
(f) to those who will be required to act on results of the test;
(g) to those who will finance the operation.

In addition, the proposed test should be *reliable*:

(a) it measures what it is meant to measure;
(b) the same result is obtained when the test is repeated, i.e. test–retest reliability;
(c) the same result is obtained when the test is done by a different examiner, i.e. inter-observer reliability;
(d) the same result is obtained when the test is done by an alternative reliable method, i.e. split sample reliability.

The proposed test should also be *valid*, i.e. the results of the test should correlate with the presence of the disorder. The relationship between test result and diagnosis can be analysed statistically, as shown in Table 12.1.

Table 12.1 Analysis of screening

(a) test positive, disorder present	(b) test positive, disorder not present	(a) + (b) all persons with positive test
(c) test negative, disorder present	(d) test negative, disorder not present	(c) + (d) all persons with negative test
(a) + (c) all persons with disorder	(b) + (d) all persons without disorder	(a) + (b) + (c) + (d) all persons tested

(a) = True positive.
(b) = False positive – if high, leads to undesirable over-referral.
(c) = False negative – 'missed' cases, may inhibit further testing.
(d) = True negative.

A satisfactory test has a high proportion of true results (i.e. a+d/a+b+c+d) and a low proportion of false results (i.e. b+c/a+b+c+d). The *sensitivity* of a test is its accuracy in correctly identifying all individuals with the disorder (i.e. a/a+c).

The *specificity* of a test is its accuracy in correctly identifying all individuals without the disorder (i.e. d/b+d).

Developmental practice

There are no short cuts or quick tests in satisfactory developmental practice. To be able to give a reliable opinion that a child is normal, to make a sound developmental diagnosis and to provide acceptable developmental guidance, personnel must be well trained.

Paediatricians are alerted to the possibility of abnormalities by listening to parents, health visitors, teachers and anyone else in contact with the child, and also by their own observations every time they have a chance to see the child. In addition, they may arrange to examine all the babies and young children in their practice at certain selected ages. The advantages of this kind of service when it is well developed are considerable:

(a) contact with the parents and observation of the child is not left to chance;
(b) some items may only come to light in this way;
(c) opportunity is provided to give developmental guidance.

From these activities, children are identified for further examination and developmental diagnosis.

Developmental diagnosis

Developmental diagnosis is based upon six items:

(a) delay in developmental pattern;
(b) distortion of developmental pattern;
(c) quantitative changes;
(d) quality of performance;
(e) application of abilities;
(f) other signs.

Delay in developmental pattern

A lot happens quickly in the first year and the characteristic developmental picture changes every few weeks. Consequently delayed development should be detected fairly easily. Consider the situation of a baby whose development is 25% behind normal expectations. This is equivalent to a week behind at 1 month, 6 weeks at 6 months, and 3 months at 1 year. It is not easy to be certain about a week's delay at 1 month of age, although suspicions may be raised if the baby seems to be unusually limp and to make insufficient attempts to raise his head. By 6 months there should be little difficulty because the infant will behave more like a 'typical' 4½ month old. Thus, full head control will have been acquired only recently and the head may still be insecure when the trunk is shaken; voluntary reaching will be just developing and transfer will not be seen; when held upright, there will be little support from the legs; and chewing actions will not be seen. An infant of 1 year showing a 25% delay of development will show actions considered to be typical of a 9 month old.

The greater the delay in development, the more serious it is. Lesser degrees of delay may not even be abnormal, but represent normal variations. It must always be remembered that the various developmental features do not appear at precisely the same age in all children; in some they occur earlier and in other cases later than the average age. In any group of normal children each individual ability appears over an age range, as illustrated in Figure 12.1. The duration of this range varies considerably with different abilities. In some cases the range is quite small. In other words, only a short time elapses between the first appearance of the particular ability in a few children and its manifestation by all children (curve A in Figure 12.1). In other cases the range may be much longer (curve B). In the case of each ability, the age at which a few children first show that particular ability can be called the 'initial age'. The age at which the majority of children show the ability is the 'limit age'. The 'mean age' is the age at which 50% of the normal popuation manifest the particular ability. These terms are used as shown below.

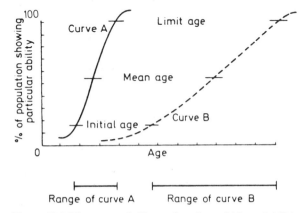

Figure 12.1 Diagrammatic illustration of acquisition of abilities showing initial, mean and limit ages, and range of abilities

Initial age
It is possible to use the concept of an 'initial age' to say of a child that his performance is comparable to the initial age level. This gives a minimal developmental age level. For example, suppose that a particular ability has an initial age of 5 months, a mean age of 7 months and a limit age of 9 months: when that ability is observed it is possible to say that the child's developmental level is *at least* 5 months.

This method is especially useful in the examination of handicapped children. It may not be possible to carry out a full examination and the clinical picture may be dominated by the child's limited abilities, but it may be possible to note a few items which can be given a minimum initial age level.

A list of initial ages for various abilities has been compiled mostly from the writings of Gesell and Amatruda (1969) and Griffiths (1967) (Table 12.2). This is not a complete list, but could provide a basis for a paediatrician's own personal list which he will tend to build up automatically as he becomes more experienced in developmental work.

Limit age
The concept of 'limit age' is used most often in quick developmental checks of normal children to detect those who require fuller examination. In these

Table 12.2 Initial ages for various childhood abilities

Age	Ability, observation of which indicates a minimum developmental age level	Age	Ability, observation of which indicates a developmental age level
1 mth	Regards object in line of vision and follows for short distances Immobilizes to nearby sound and social approach Prone, raises head just clear of table	1 yr	Gives a toy; releases cube into cup Co-operates with dressing Walks one hand held Responds to 'No' and 'Give it'
4 mth	Very slight head lag when pulled to sitting Almost complete head stability in sitting Prompt visual regard Holds ring, reaches for it with free hand and takes it to mouth	1½ yr	Sits down on chair Builds tower of 4–5 cubes Spontaneous scribble Looks at picture book and may name or point to one picture Carries doll or teddy and hugs it Obeys simple directions
6 mth	Immediate reach for object and retention in radial palmar grasp Transfers object (cube) from hand to hand Sits momentarily on a firm surface Takes feet to mouth Discriminates strangers	2 yr	Towers 6–7 cubes Imitates vertical stroke and circle Names pictures (2 or 3) Kicks ball Follows directions Walks up and down stairs
9 mth	Index finger approach to small objects Early pincer grasp Shakes bell Pulls objects towards himself with string Pulls to standing Pat-a-cakes (claps hands) and waves 'Bye bye' Imitates sounds and uses 'Mama', 'Dada' with meaning	3 yr	With book turns pages singly and names pictures With crayon early tripod grip, copies circle and names drawing Asks questions: may answer one or two Knows name and sex Repeats up to 3 digits Matches 3 colours

circumstances, any child who is not showing abilities when beyond the limit age for those abilities (i.e. beyond the age when the majority of children show the particular ability) should be identified and examined. Unlike the concept of initial age, which can be applied to both what Gesell and Amatruda called 'permanent' and 'temporary' abilities, the concept of limit age can be applied in developmental diagnosis only to permanent abilities.

Gesell and Amatruda had something similar to limit age tests in mind when they presented their list of the latest ages for acceptable appearance of certain abilities. Egan, Illingworth and MacKeith (1969) and Sheridan (1973), in describing the developmental examination of the young child, listed several items at each age the absence of which made it mandatory to investigate further. Neligan and Prudham (1969) also introduced the idea of upper age limits for certain simple items which members of a primary medical care team – health visitor and general practitioner – could use in order to pick out those children in need of further examination. From these and various other sources a list of limit age tests has been devised (Table 12.3). It must be emphasized that this concept of limit age tests is a clinical one to assist developmental paediatricians when there is only a little time available for the

Table 12.3 Limit ages for various childhood abilities

Age (mth)	Ability which should be shown by stated age (if absent or doubtful, further examination is indicated)
1	Some indication of attention
2	Attention to objects Some response to nearby voices and everyday noises
3	Head held erect
4	Hands not fisted Shows ordinary interest in people and playthings
5	Reaches for object
6	ATNR* not present or producible Visual fixation and following established Turns to sounds
7	Holds objects in hands
9	Gives attention to gestures
10	Sits independently on firm surfaces Uses tuneful babble to self and others Bears most of weight on legs Chews lumpy food
12	Attends to words
15	Releases held object
18	Walks alone No casting, mouthing, drooling
21	Kicks when standing Says single words with meaning
27	Puts 2–3 words together into a phrase
3 yr	Can stand on one leg Talks in sentences
4 yr	Uses fully intelligible speech

* ATNR, asymmetric tonic neck reflex

examination. Not all children selected for further examination in this way will be abnormal; examples can be quoted of children who were remarkably late in various skills and yet turned out to be normal (Illingworth, 1972), and conversely some of the individuals not selected by limit age tests will be abnormal and these children will be detected in most cases by observing an abnormal or poor quality of performance.

As an illustration of the application of initial and limit ages, we may consider the case of a 20-month-old child who is taken to see a paediatrician because of failure to walk. This is beyond the limit age for walking (18 months), and he must be fully investigated and considered to be abnormal until proven otherwise. If the child is responsive to simple commands and will give a cube to the examiner on request, the developmental level is at least 12 months because this is the initial age for these items. This child therefore requires an exploration of developmental abilities between 12 and 18 months.

Mean age

The 'mean age' is used in most psychological tests as the age level basis for scoring the test. The use of standard deviations along with the mean age is useful. The initial age corresponds to approximately 2 SD below the mean age, and the limit age to approximately 2 SD above.

Distortion of developmental pattern

Everyone who studies child development soon becomes aware of the smooth integration which normally exists between the various features, and when this pattern is distorted the more likely is it that an abnormality is present. Nevertheless, variations are frequently seen which are not due to any abnormality and they should not be labelled and treated as if they were. Developmental paediatricians need to be aware of these normal variations, in order to protect infants from wrongful diagnoses and to be able to give sound developmental guidance to parents.

Quite considerable variations occur in behaviour. Mothers soon recognize that their baby has a characteristic personality. If their baby is very different from others, for example if he is exceptionally irritable, they will need to be reassured that he is perfectly well and normal, assuming that examinations show this to be so, and they will need guidance about his rearing.

Interesting variations occur with respect to infants' responses to visual and auditory stimuli; whereas most infants learn to respond to both types of stimuli, some infants develop an intense fascination for one or the other. This is usually a temporary phase; but it may last several months, and during this time the infants' behaviour is influenced by his particular sensory preference.

Considerable variations of motor activity occur normally in the first year. Rearing patterns influence infants' motor performance in the early months, as shown by the fact that it is possible to distinguish babies who spend most of their time in the prone position from those who spend most of their time supine (Holt, 1960). Babies who are placed prone for most of the time from birth onwards behave more confidently in the prone position and appear to be advanced for their age. They soon begin to 'scoot' – an activity in which they push or pull themselves with their hands and so begin to move about in the prone position – and later they often favour crawling for mobility and use this for quite a long time. In contrast, their performance in the supine position and when pulled to sitting appears to be immature, inept and delayed when compared with the performance of babies who spend most of their time in a supine position. These early posturally induced variations of motor performance do not appear to have a lasting effect upon other aspects of development.

Robson (1984) has made some particularly interesting studies of early motor development. He describes normal variations in which prolonged crawling and bottom-shuffling are the principal means of mobility. He considers that familial influences are important in these cases because a history of similar variant patterns is obtained from other members of the family. These variations do affect later development. Independent walking, for example, occurs later than usual. He suggests that late onset of walking should not be considered to be abnormal in these cases of unusual motor development without other evidence.

Quantitative changes

Observing the quantitative aspects of behaviour is useful. Does the infant spend too little time on tasks? This might be abnormal. Does the infant spend a lot of time on any particular task? This might be acceptable and normal if the particular activity was acquired recently and is appropriate for his age. Too much interest upon one activity at the expense of other activities is as worrying as too little interest in anything. For example, hand regard is commonly seen at about 5 months of age. Much of this activity might be considered useful if it lasted only a week or two, because during that time it could indicate reinforcement of eye–hand co-ordination. Its persistence for a long period and its presence at a later age should, however, alert one to the possibility of abnormality, for why otherwise should this action be long continued and not replaced by something more constructive?

Quality of performance

Paediatricians obtain many useful clues from noting the quality of performance of children as they carry out various tasks during a developmental examination. The information obtained in this way enables them to detect a number of children with developmental problems who would otherwise not be noted until much later. The paediatricians' medical, especially neurological, training is invaluable to them in this respect.

The items noted by an alert paediatrician include the following:

the child's composure;
the ease and smoothness of the child's movements;
the normality of his posture in standing and sitting;
his attentiveness and concentration;
the promptness of his comprehension and responsiveness;
the presence of tremor or ataxia, especially during manipulative tasks;
unusual posturing of the hands when carrying out a task;
evidence of excessive muscle action;
the presence of mirror movements;
difficulties brought to light when the child is asked to increase the speed or accuracy
    of performance;
poor eye–hand co-ordination;
the use of trick movements.

Application of abilities

The paediatrician should observe what use the infant makes of every stimulus he perceives and every action he performs. Suspicion is immediately raised in the case of any infant who fails to make use of his opportunities. If an infant can reach out to take hold of objects, does he do so? And what does he do when he has got the objects? If an infant can roll, does he indulge in this activity randomly or does he use this motor skill to get from place to place, or to reach his toys? Constructive use of activities is an encouraging feature.

Other signs

A developmental paediatrician's great asset is his ability to use information from his general examination in the interpretation of his developmental observations.

For example, in the case of an infant showing minor developmental variations, he will view these more seriously if he also finds in his general examination variations of muscle strength and tone and tendon reflexes.

Developmental guidance

Developmental guidance (Holt, 1979) is valuable for all parents and carers of children, whether the children are normal or not. Several types of guidance exist, as described below.

Reassurance

Rearing a small child is a demanding task. Many parents are anxious and worry about minor problems. Cox, Zinkin and Grimsby (1974) found that over one-third of mothers attending child development clinics were worried even when all was well with their child. Richman (1976) found that over 40% of mothers suffered depression as a result of child-rearing anxieties. The situation is aggravated by the fragmentation and dispersal of families which occurs at the present time. Reassurance may seem old fashioned and a long way from scientific medicine, but it can make a lot of difference to many parents.

Explanatory

Many parents do not understand why their child does what he or she does. As a result they miss a lot of enjoyment of their child; they do not help the child as often and as well as they could; and they may even punish the child unreasonably. Time spent on explanatory developmental guidance increases their interest in the child and also makes them more sensitive to his needs and responses. The phenomenon of casting provides a good example. Casting occurs early in the second year. Toys, food, shoes, socks and any other suitable object may be played with for a little while and then thrown away, often over the side of the cot, pram or high-chair. Some mothers despair. How can they keep the home tidy? How can they teach their child to be less troublesome? It has to be explained that this behaviour is both normal and desirable. It is normal because it is shown by almost all children at this early age. It is desirable because it occurs shortly after infants become aware of the continued existence of objects once they leave their hands. Casting seems to reinforce that understanding, almost as if the child is proving to himself that what he has in his hand also exists when he throws it to the floor. The action also gives the child a sense of distance and space. When a mother appreciates these points she no longer scolds her child for untidiness, but picks up the toys with a smile and makes the occasion one of pleasant play and interaction. Explanatory developmental guidance promotes first of all understanding and then confidence.

Reinforcing

Encouraging a child's useful and desirable actions never comes amiss and always pays good dividends. It may take the form of praise when he has completed something, or helping him to complete a task at just the moment he begins to give up.

Inhibiting

Undesirable behaviour and action have to be controlled and parents need advice about the ways to do so. All too often they react forcefully and may then actually reinforce rather than inhibit the particular behaviour.

Co-ordinating

When some aspect of development is out of step with others, the deviant behaviour can be very troublesome. An attempt has to be made to correct the problem and to restore an integrated pattern of development. For example, the hearing impaired girl in Figure 12.2 has to watch faces to fully understand what is being said. Doing so takes her attention away from her hands and disturbs the development of eye–hand co-ordination. Her mother needs to be made aware of the situation and encouraged to allow her daughter to look at both her face and her own hands.

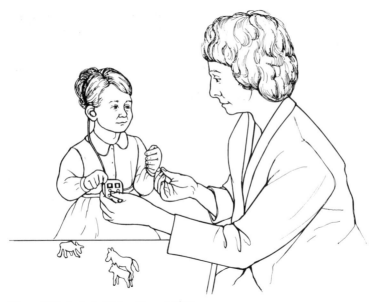

Figure 12.2 A deaf child and her mother

Anticipating

It is surprising how often parents of first children are unaware of the stages of development. They are ill-prepared for what comes next. Their 7 month old was spontaneously happy with everyone. Now at 10 months he cries when their neighbour visits. They see it as a problem and a deterioration of his behaviour, but really his behaviour has changed because he is now more aware of strangers and the different characters of people he meets. This is a normal developmental advance which is seen as a problem, but it need not be so if parents receive anticipatory guidance.

In the case of children with problems, developmental guidance is continued and linked with therapeutic advice and counselling.

References

Alberman, E. D. and Goldstein, H. (1970) The 'at risk' register: a statistical evaluation. *Br. J. Prev. Soc. Med.*, **24**, 129–135

Butler, J. (1989) *Child Health Surveillance in Primary Care*. London: HMSO

Cox, C. A., Zinkin, P. M. and Grimsby, M. F. J. (1974) Aspects of the six month developmental examination in a longitudinal study. *Devl. Med. Child Neurol.*, **19**, 149–159

Egan, D., Illingworth, R. S. and MacKeith, R. C. (1969) Developmental screening 0–5 years. *Clinics Dev. Med. 30*. London: Heinemann

Frankenberg, W. K. (1974) Selection of diseases and tests in paediatric screening. *Pediatrics*, **54**, 612–616

Gesell, A. and Amatruda, C. S. (1969) *Developmental Diagnosis*. New York: Harper and Row

Griffiths, R. (1967) *The Abilities of Babies*, 4th edn. London: University of London Press

Hall, D. M. B. (1988) *Health for all Children*. Oxford: Oxford University Press

Holt, K. S. (1960) Early motor development: posturally induced variations. *J. Pediat.*, **57**, 571

Holt, K. S. (1979) Development guidance. *Child Care Hlth Dev.* **5**, 249

Illingworth, R. S. (1972) *The Development of the Infant and Young Child – Normal and Abnormal*. Edinburgh: Churchill Livingstone

Neligan, G. and Prudham, D. (1969) Potential value of four early developmental milestones in screening children for increased risk of later retardation. *Devl. Med. Child Neurol.*, **11**, 423

Richman, N. (1976) Depression in mothers of pre-school children. *J. Child Psychol. Psychiat.*, **17**, 75–78

Robson, P. (1984) Pre-walking locomotor movements and their use in predicting standing and walking. *Child Care Hlth Dev.*, **10**, 317

Sheridan, M. D. (1973) *Children's Developmental Progress*. Windsor: NFER

Chapter 13

A developmental approach to handicapped children

Promoting the development of the handicapped child

When paediatricians encounter any child showing abnormal development, or any condition which might interfere with his development, they should strive to find out all they can about the conditions and then try to promote the child's development. Their efforts should be along the following principal directions:

(a) conveying an understanding of the child's development and his limitations to all who are concerned with him;
(b) reinforcing the child's most recently acquired abilities and ensuring that they are used most productively;
(c) providing missed experiences;
(d) making use of other skills possessed by the child to overcome his difficulties;
(e) using external means, e.g. aids, appliances and toys, at an appropriate developmental level to overcome the child's difficulties.

Conveying an understanding of a child's development and limitations

This is best done by example. If we show our understanding of a child's development by the way we do things with him and to him, it will be noticed by parents and others and then copied by them. To be able to do this, it is necessary to be able to size up the child's developmental level quickly and to make approaches to him at that level. It is also most essential to be sensitive to the child's reactions. The following extract from the discussion of child–stranger encounters by Tinbergen and Tinbergen (1972) reveals the insensitiveness of our usual contacts with children:

> When meeting a child . . . the observer . . . either smiles or simply looks at the child. Its responses are extremely varied. They can range from, on the one hand, definitely positive to, on the other, gaze aversion, and closing of the eyes, turning of the head, and even of the whole body, and snuggling up against the mother. . . . Between these extremes there are numerous intermediate response patterns, some of them extremely subtle – so subtle in fact that, although one can learn to recognize them at a glance, one has to make a quite intense analysis of one's own perception before one can make explicit what one has actually seen. . . . the child . . . can show various types of friendly, socially positive behaviour; subtle expressions of the eyes and body stance which one learns to recognize as, for instance, interested, or friendly, etc.; very slight curving up of the corners of the mouth; continued eye contact, etc. . . . The initial, exploratory glance can on other

occasions be followed by a negative response pattern. . . . The mildest expression of a rejecting attitude is a certain expression of the eyes . . . the response of the adult to this first stage of the child's behaviour has in turn a powerful communicative effect on the child. . . . These sequences, very obvious once one has observed them, are often overlooked because, as a rule, this happens so quickly, and because most of us react unconsciously by looking away ourselves, and so see no more than the child's first response.

Conveying an understanding of a child's development may take the form of explaining to his parents why a child behaves in the way he does. For example, parents may complain that their young child ignores them when they speak to him while he is playing at the further side of the room. They fear he may be deaf. Careful hearing tests show that there is no hearing impairment at all. At this stage they are usually 'reassured' and dismissed, but this does not solve their problem. Parents' worries should not be dismissed as due to fussiness and anxiety. They want to know why their child is behaving as he does. Perhaps in this particular case it was because he became mobile before he was quite ready to do so from the point of view of auditory development, and he cannot yet maintain auditory awareness at a distance. Consequently if the parents are encouraged to move nearer to him and get his attention before speaking, they will find he will respond to them.

Recommendations should be explained. For example, when a young child has to be admitted to hospital we always recommend that his mother should stay with him because young children do not have an understanding of time and to be apart from his mother may seem to the child that she has gone altogether. And again, it may seem strange to recommend to a mother of a deaf and blind child that she wear the same perfume each day – what has this to do with medicine? In fact it is vitally important that such an afflicted child receive every possible clue to his surroundings. The perfume becomes for him a familiar and constant signal from the outside world. Such children panic when the perfume is changed.

It is important to convey an understanding of a child's development to his parents in all cases. Some parents feel to be all at sea with even completely normal babies, but when there is something wrong they are quite lost and do not know what to expect. They need to know what they can do with regard to handling their child and administering discipline and stimulation. We find that it is very useful to give parents a report of developmental progress each time their child is re-examined. Developmental guidance is given at this time, as illustrated by the following example.

Peter is a 3½-year-old physically well-developed boy who shows considerable delay in all his abilities, and his 'developmental level' lies between 14 and 16 months. His parents do not realize the limitations of such a physically active child with whom they constantly have battles because he does not do what they expect him to be able to do. They bought him a small tricycle which he ignores, and many other toys such as model cars and stuffed animals, but he does not play with them for very long and he treats them roughly, often throwing them on the floor.

What should they expect and what should they do? Peter is mobile, but he has few abilities to make constructive use of this mobility. He will use his mobility to explore, but he is unlikely to find anything to hold his interest for long. He is likely to move about apparently aimlessly, seeming to have a short span of attention and being easily distracted. If this situation continues he is likely to increase his mobility even further and could go on to the full picture of 'hyperactivity'. They should try to make his movements as interesting as possible and try to arrange that there is something to hold his attention, however briefly, at appropriate intervals. Even trying to hold his attention for a short spell will help to prevent the development of valueless hyperactivity.

Peter is not yet at the stage of development when he can understand symbolic representation. So his toys are all objects and he treats them accordingly. He is at the stage of exploring the inside and outside of objects, so for play materials he needs boxes into which he can put and take out other objects. He cannot yet make use of the more sophisticated toys he has been given, but he can be given more visual, auditory and tactile stimulation at his present level of play, e.g. boxes of different textures, and colours and designs, and some of them capable of producing sounds.

So far as language is concerned he is still at the stage of needing much input which should consist of appropriate verbal stimulation nearby. But what does this mean? Just because he is moving about all the time and apparently showing little interest is no reason to stop talking to him. His parents are advised to move towards him, and to get his attention and then to speak to him as clearly as possible. Because his attention is short and he only has concepts of concrete objects, the verbal stimulation should be short and concerned with definite objects which Peter should be able to see and touch. For example, 'Peter, ball; this is the ball; Peter have the ball.' Here his attention is first caught by calling his name, then he is immediately shown the ball so that he mentally focuses upon the object, then several short phrases are used in which the key word 'ball' is repeated frequently.

Discipline is not easy at this stage. Although Peter's parents may feel that at 3½ years of age he is a big boy and should behave better than he does, he is just not ready to do so. He is at a developmental stage in which periods of resistance and tantrums are quite common. The more his parents try to overcome this, the more tantrums they are likely to precipitate. Use should be made of his easy distractability, and when he does some undesired action he should be distracted onto some other task.

All this may seem very obvious, but it is extremely difficult for parents to take a new look at their own child and to begin to appreciate his real level of functioning. These basic developmental issues may have to be discussed with them many times.

Reinforcing the child's recently acquired abilities and facilitating their productive use

Normal healthy children may often be seen practising their recently acquired abilities. It seems to give them considerable pleasure and satisfaction. This practice is useful because it helps to improve the skill of performance and ensures its establishment in the child's repertoire of abilities. When development is delayed or distorted, however, such spontaneous practice and reinforcement does not seem to occur as frequently. Consequently, new abilities are often very frail and tenuous and there is a risk that they may not persist. If, in these circumstances, the newest abilities are pointed out to parents they will be able to play often with the child to provide the necessary practice. The following is an example of this type of developmental guidance taken from one of the case records of a deaf child.

> He demonstrates good object-recognition by using everyday objects appropriately and is just beginning to get an understanding of symbols, therefore extending his communication range from his present 'direct' system to a simple (pre-language) symbol system for

everyday events. For example, put the brush and some other object in front of him, gesture hair-brushing at the same time as saying the word, and reward appropriate responses. He now appreciates personal rewards such as a kiss or clapped hands.

The reinforcement of the very earliest step in the development of symbolization described above is recommended in order to establish this ability and so enable the child to be able to use it for further steps forward.

Providing missed experiences

Disabled children frequently miss out on experiences and learning opportunities which other children enjoy, so it is desirable to provide them with additional experiences to offset their developmental limitations. For example, a child who lacks mobility after the first year is greatly limited. As he cannot move around to explore, it may be possible to arrange for him to be able to get things to go to him. A useful device for such an immobile child is a small chest on castors which he can pull towards him with a piece of string in order to explore its contents (Figure 13.1).

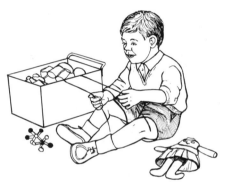

Figure 13.1 Overcoming immobility to get exploration experiences

One mother's account of the response to her daughter's first experience of independent mobility provided through an electric-powered chair vividly revealed the importance of the new experiences. Her daughter was 4 years of age and was severely disabled by athetoid cerebral palsy. Her intelligence was good, but she could not move about and so was totally dependent on others coming to her and moving her from place to place. Placed in a powered chair, she soon mastered the controls and could move about as she wished. Her mother called her for lunch and she moved away down the garden path – the first display of normal impishness her mother had ever encountered. She played hide and seek with her brothers and sisters in the garden. Even indoors she moved around in her chair and surprised her parents by sudden appearances. Her joy with this sudden wealth of experiences showed how much she had been missing.

In various ways, children who miss out on early learning experiences can be helped by being given comparable opportunities. Every child with developmental delay or distortion should be studied to determine what he is missing and what can be done to replace the lost experiences.

Making use of other skills possessed by the child to overcome his difficulties

Sometimes it is possible to use one ability to overcome difficulties due to the limitation of other abilities. Perhaps the best example is when a child's verbal abilities are fairly well developed and are used to assist his performance, and to overcome visuo-motor problems. The child is shown how to identify differences between objects and to verbalize these differences so that he can carry out some action. He may have failed a formboard test, but succeeds when he has learnt to say to himself: 'This has a corner here and here and should fit into this hole.'

Using external means at an appropriate developmental level

The whole subject of the use of aids and appliances to assist handicapped children is beyond the scope of this present volume. One special group of aids, however, deserves special mention. These are toys.

By careful selection, toys can be particularly useful for handicapped children (Riddick, 1982). Highly expensive and 'special' toys are not necessary. The important thing is their proper selection and appropriate use. The following are examples of toys especially useful in the case of certain disabilities.

Toys for a handicapped child unable to move about (vision and hands normal)

Mental age	Requirements
Up to 6 months	Similar to a normal baby. Nearby toys to look at, to reach for and hold in palm; to explore with two hands; to take to mouth. Safety important.
6–12 months	Toys to stimulate developing skills of index-finger poking, finger–thumb grasp, grasp and release, squeezing. Toys similar to those needed for normal child of this age, but, because the child is not mobile, various devices must be used to bring the toys into the child's range, e.g. trays, peg or magnetic boards fitted to side of pram or cot, hanging toys. Suggested toys: box to put things into and to take out, finger-flicking toys, wheels, squeezy toys, musical strings to pluck, paper, bendy toys.
1–3 years	A time when normal children are very active exploring and getting many new and recurring experiences. Needs: pictures and models to reinforce impressions, simple fitting toys, simple puzzle toys, e.g. boxes with different types of fastenings, adjacent locker, threading toys, different materials, e.g. clay, sand, simple building blocks.

3–5+ years	Similar to previous period, but more advanced and more imitative of daily activities. Larger sizes. Not always toys but sometimes the real objects. Simple construction tasks lasting up to 10–15 min. Doll's house.

Toys as walking aids

Solid firm objects which allow child to pull himself to standing.	Small, solid, fixed table and chairs, wall bars frame.
To provide support in walking.	Pushing toys must be sufficiently weighted not to tip, and be of adjustable height, with hand-holds of various types appropriate to the hand function.
To motivate movement whether as crawling or walking.	Pushing, pulling, rolling and mechanical toys, e.g. balls, toys on wheels, skittles.

Toys to stimulate various hand functions

Grasp (palmar).	Small balls, squeezy toys, blocks, clay.
Grasp (finger–thumb).	Threading beads, peg-board, small construction toys, chalk, pencils, small models, e.g. farms, doll's house, soldiers to pick up, pulling toys.
Index finger use.	Pointing and pressing actions, cash register, telephone, finger-flicking toys, large clock.
Supination of hand.	Carrying tray or large box, toys with large handles needing clockwise rotation for right hand and anticlockwise for left hand, large balls, toys working only on upward pressure with palm of hand.
Bilateral hand use (both hands).	Large balls, large boxes, rolling pins, building jars, barrels, eggs, drums, xylophone, stirring, threading, winding, screwing toys, barrel organ.
Individual finger use.	Sewing, knitting, piano, clay modelling, scissors.

Adjustments to toys for the child with poor vision
Avoid toys which are too small to be seen clearly and those with small parts and patterns.
  Use toys which stimulate tactile impressions, e.g. different textures and shapes.

Adjustments to toys for the child with poor hearing
Use toys which produce a variety of different sounds.

Toys to stimulate space perception
Toys consisting of simple shapes to fit together.
Toys fitting into one another.

Toys encouraging exploration of areas, e.g. toy sweeping brush, doll's furniture.
Toys needing hanging on hooks, etc.
Pouring from jars and buckets with water and sand.
Drawing and painting both on flat surfaces and of objects, e.g. wooden boxes.

Additional information about toys and developmental play is available from the Toy Libraries Association (Toynbee Hall, 28 Commercial Street, London E1 6LS).

Developmental approach to cerebral palsy

The developmental approach to the management and training of handicapped children will be further illustrated by reference to one particular group of disabilities – cerebral palsy.

First it is necessary to appreciate that the relationship and interactions between mother and child are seldom normal. The mother is extremely anxious about her baby. Events during pregnancy or delivery, such as episodes of bleeding, premature labour or severe asphyxia, make her particularly sensitive about the progress of the baby, and many mothers are aware that all is not well with their baby some time before a diagnosis is established. The baby often appears to have been rendered especially sensitive and vulnerable as a result of the neurological lesion. These two aspects interact and reinforce each other. The tenseness and irritability of the baby makes the mother more anxious, and her greater anxiety is reflected in even more tenseness and irritability on the part of the baby. A vicious spiral effect results. These events are shown diagrammatically in Figure 13.2.

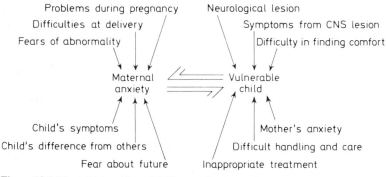

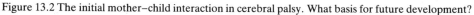

Figure 13.2 The initial mother–child interaction in cerebral palsy. What basis for future development?

Our experiences suggest that some of the clinical features observed in babies with cerebral palsy are due to this vicious spiral interaction effect. The first step therefore is to reduce and to reverse it, which is done by showing an understanding of the child's problems and the mother's difficulties; by discussing the symptoms and signs; and by showing how the baby can be examined and handled. As the mother loses a little of her anxiety, she can be encouraged to carry out some of the everyday tasks which have been frightening her, such as picking up her baby, and feeding him. When she finds she can now do this without the previous difficulties, her confidence begins to return. In this way the vicious spiral of interaction is reversed. These initial steps need to be handled with great sensitivity. When this is done satisfactorily some of the infant's symptoms subside, his mother gains confidence and can actively contribute to the next developmental stages, and a firm basis is established for later treatment.

Too hasty action at this early stage, such as by simply attaching a diagnostic label and referring for therapy, aggravates the situation by confirming the mother's fears that her baby is abnormal, and her feeling of inadequacy because a professional worker now has to do things to her baby.

Problems and anxieties arise in the rearing of healthy babies, but there exists a ready source of interest and advice from friends, neighbours and relatives, and without this support mothers feel isolated and uncertain. In the case of babies with developmental problems, the friends, neighbours and relatives cannot help because *their* babies were normal. Parents of babies with problems need advice and help from those who understand the situation – the professional workers and parents of other affected children.

The next step is to make a very detailed review of the infant's care throughout each 24 hours. This review often reveals other maternal anxieties which may not otherwise have come to light. For example, did she buy the best cot for him; does she keep the room temperature correct; what should she do when he suddenly thrusts backwards? These items are discussed as they arise.

As the 24-hour review is carried out, it is possible to indicate more effective ways of doing various things so as to cause less distress to the child and also to promote his progress and development. For example, the hip adductor muscles may be unusually tight and it is considered desirable to stretch them in order to safeguard the stability of the hip joints. This can be achieved by showing the mother how the baby can be carried with his legs spread either side of the mother's hip and ensuring that this position is adopted every time he is carried. In this way, useful measures are incorporated quite simply and effectively into the everyday care of the child, whereas if abduction of the hips was done in a treatment session it would add to the day's work and disrupt normal routine.

The 'informal therapy' introduced during the 24-hour review may cover the child's needs, but if more specialized 'formal therapy' is indicated, a good basis for it has been provided.

All treatment, whether in special sessions or in the everyday routine, includes the following principles.

In most cases it is necessary to strive to overcome the persistence of early reflex activities. There are good reasons for attempting to reduce persisting and excessive reflex activities. Their persistence delays both general development and motor development; it may also lead to deformity; and it may become a self-perpetuating movement ritual. Treatment consists of finding out the factors which precipitate the excessive activity and, if possible, eliminating them; finding the postures which reduce the reflex activity, and here a treatment system such as that developed by Bobath and Bobath (1957) can be useful (Figure 13.3); and by the judicious use of drugs such as diazepam (valium) (Figure 13.4).

As a result of the delay of motor development and the neurological abnormalities, most children with cerebral palsy lie in one or two different postures. They find it particularly difficult to change their posture and to get into and maintain any anti-gravity posture. There are several major consequences of these difficulties. The failure to develop head control against gravity delays auditory localization and impedes visual exploration of the surroundings, and it

Spontaneous activity   In reflex inhibiting posture
at rest

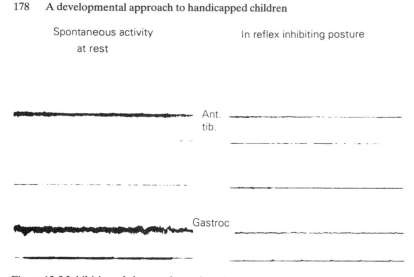

Figure 13.3 Inhibition of abnormal muscle activity by Bobath technique

also makes feeding difficult. Impairment of head control and poor arm movements delays the development of eye–hand co-ordination which is so essential for the later development of many motor skills. Deformities are particular liable to occur if the child stays in the same posture for long periods. So there are a good number of reasons, many related to the child's developmental needs, for ensuring that cerebral-palsied children are placed in many different postures and are stimulated to acquire anti-gravity postures. The components of early motor development are stimulated and practised in several treatment systems (e.g. Cotton, 1974). At the same time, while in these various postures, the child is encouraged to make the fullest possible use of his learning opportunities. For example, visual and auditory localization, eye–hand co-ordination and reaching are practised.

Mobility is a most important aspect of early child development (Holt, 1975). Children use movement for their own pleasure, exploration, communication, and the elaboration of emotional relationships. For many children with cerebral palsy, mobility does not develop at the appropriate time, so some form of movement, either passive or active, has to be provided to overcome the detrimental effects of immobility such as deprivation of learning opportunities. To mention just one example, we have found that electrically powered chairs have opened up new worlds for quite young cerebral-palsied children.

It soon becomes necessary to promote mother–child emancipation. The mother's natural reaction to her handicapped child and all the extra things she does for him increases mother and child dependence in the early stages, but this situation cannot be allowed to continue for too long. This severance does not occur spontaneously, as in the course of normal development, but has to be arranged. The immobile child cannot physically wean himself from his mother as a normal child does when he slips from her knee and crawls across the floor. If the early steps described above were achieved with her full understanding, the need to sever this bond will be appreciated by the mother. The handling of this situation is one of the most difficult, delicate and important tasks for anyone caring for the young cerebral-palsied child, and it requires much help and guidance.

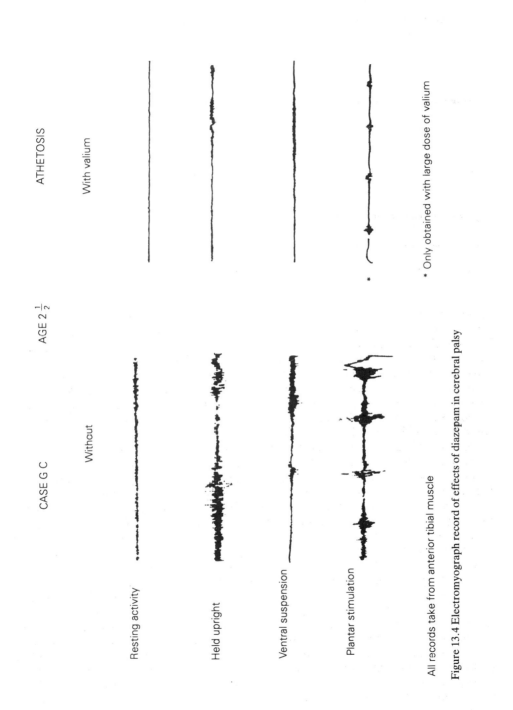

Figure 13.4 Electromyograph record of effects of diazepam in cerebral palsy

References

Bobath, B. and Bobath, K. (1957) Control of motor function in the treatment of cerebral palsy. *Physiotherapy, Lond.,* October

Cotton, E. (1974) Improvement in motor function with the use of conductive education. *Devl. Med. Child Neurol.,* **16,** 637

Holt, K. S. (1975) Movement and child development. *Clinics Child Dev.* **55**, London: Heinemann

Riddick, B. (1982) *Toys and Play for the Handicapped Child.* London: Croom Helm

Tinbergen, E. A. and Tinbergen, N. (1972) *Early Childhood Autism – An Ethological Approach.* Berlin: Parey

Chapter 14

Measures of development

Measurement is the basis of all science, and with regard to child development is required as a guide to progress and estimation of the extent of deviation from the normal.

Many procedures have been described. Some are simple, but others are complex and can be used only after appropriate training: some measure several abilities and attempt to present an overall measure of development and intelligence, whereas others explore specific areas.

Paediatricians need to know about these measurements not only because they may use some themselves, but so as to be able to understand and evaluate the reports of tests used by psychologists, speech therapists and other professionals. They have to decide the significance of the tests and will ask themselves questions such as:

What does the child have to do in the test?
What age range does it cover?
How long does the test last?
Will it be affected by motor, visual, auditory or visual disabilities?
How reliable is it?
Just what does it tell one about the child?

Tests and measurements complement diagnosis and are not a substitute for it. On their own they are incomplete and they have to be evaluated in the light of a carefully taken history and thorough clinical appraisal.

Some of the more frequently used procedures are described below.

Objective observation

Observation methods which were devised for research studies can be applied also to everyday clinical practice (Holt and Reynell, 1967). Planned observation techniques require time, but not as much time as might be imagined and, as they are sometimes the only methods available to provide reliable information, the time is well spent. The circumstances in which they are particularly useful include the following:

1. In the evaluation of children who will not co-operate in any form of examination or test. By this means it is possible to obtain some objective information in even the most difficult cases.

Table 14.1 Dangers of inference (Holt and Reynell, 1967)

Actual observation	Observer biased towards 'autism'	Observer biased towards deafness
2.45. Pulling a chair around the floor. Snatches at B's pram. Desists when his mother says quietly 'No, Robin'. Spins a wheeled-chair. Goes back to ordinary chair, pulls it around and spins it. Spins himself. Spins wheeled-chair. Champing jaw movements all the time. Spins all chairs in turn, flaps hands	2.45. Pulling a chair around the floor. Interested only in the furniture and not people. Takes B's pram just as an object with wheels, spinning everything. Takes no notice of people. Does not go to his mother or look at her when she speaks to him	2.45. Pulling chairs around. Does not respond to the sounds of the other children, or to his mother's voice calling him
2.50. Sitting on the floor gazing at a red square. Champing jaws. Spins a chair. Climbs onto a chair and off again. His mother goes out of the room, and his behaviour does not alter. Sits on the floor. Spins a chair. Hand flapping. Quiet, monotonous vocalization	2.50. Mesmerized by the colour red on the floor. Still spinning chairs. Does not notice his mother leaving the room	2.50. Sitting on the floor. Visually absorbed. Climbs onto a chair. Does not hear his mother go out of the room. Monotonous vocalization, just like a deaf child
2.55. Still spinning chairs and champing jaws. Vocalizes a loud 'er'. Rests his face on a chair, then lies on the ground. Gets up again and spins chair. His mother goes out. Pokes his eye. Spins a chair. Screams when his mother comes in and picks him up. She takes him to the toilet where he continues to scream	2.55. Still obsessed by his spinning activities. Then tries to retreat from the world by hiding his face on a chair and then on the ground. Objects to the interruption of his activity when his mother takes him to the toilet. Panics at the strange surroundings	2.55. Still the same monotonous vocalization. Lies down for a rest. Does not hear his mother go out again. Does not hear her come up to him, so he screams when she picks him up. She cannot explain to him about the toilet, because he cannot hear words, so he continues to scream

Denver Developmental Scale (DDS) (Frankenberg and Dodds, 1968)

This scale was designed for use by paediatricians and ancillary child health personnel when they saw babies in their first year. The age ranges for a number of developmental features are shown on an easily read chart. Figure 14.1 shows a slightly modified DDS suitable for use with children in South Wales (Bryant, Davies and Newcombe, 1974). Most children will be marked in the open boxes which cover a range from the 25th to 75th centile. The cross-hatched areas extend the range of abilities to the 90th centile, so a child who has not developed a particular ability before the end of this section requires careful examination.

Developmental Scheme of Starte (1972)

Starte devised procedures for use at defined key ages in the pre-school period and introduced grading of the responses. His scheme for a 7 months examination is shown in Table 14.2.

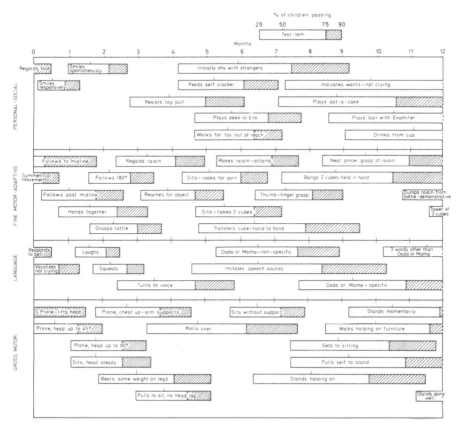

Figure 14.1 Denver Developmental Scale (Cardiff modification)

Developmental Procedure of Hooper, Curtis-Jenkins and Holt (1984)

Long experience of developmental work in general practice led Hooper and his colleagues to devise a scheme for examination at prescribed key ages which included grading of the responses and also information about the family, mother's comments, everyday abilities and the results of a physical examination. Their record card for 30 months is shown in Figure 14.2.

Other similar procedures

Often procedures are devised by paediatricians to suit their own personal practice. For example, Bellman and Cash (1987) devised a 'schedule of growing skills' for use in health districts in the UK as part of the preventative work of the community child health services, whereas Lingam (1987) had developing countries in mind when he devised his scheme.

The *Bus Puzzle test* of Egan and Brown (1984) is described in Chapter 10.

Table 14.2 Developmental screening examination at 7 months (Starte, 1972)

Test	Grade of response				
	1	2	3	4	5
Brick (cube)	No grasp	Palmar grasp	Mouthing	Transferring	Finger manipulation
Smartie (coloured sweet)	No interest	Whole hand scrabble. No pick-up	Whole hand scrabble and pick-up	Fingers and thumb pick-up	Index finger and thumb pick-up
Rattle	No interest	Transient interest and manipulation	Prolonged interest and manipulation	Manipulation and eventual imitation	Immediate imitation
Bell	No interest	Transient interest and manipulation	Prolonged interest and manipulation	Manipulation and eventual imitation	Immediate imitation
Rolling balls (Stycar)	¾ in or larger	½ in	¼ in	³⁄₁₆ in	⅛ in
6 sounds	No hearing demonstrated	Response to 1–3 sounds or marked difference between 2 sides	Slow response both sides, 4–5 sounds	Rapid response both sides, 4–5 sounds	Rapid response both sides, 6 sounds
Prone	Head up not sustained	Head up, weight on forearms	Head up, shoulders up, weight on hands	Head and shoulders up, knee up	Crawls
Sitting	No sitting stability. Hyper- or hypotonic	Sits briefly with support then unstable, back hypotonic	Sits upright, needs examiner's hand on back	Sits upright steadily, unsupported	Reaches to each side without toppling
Standing	No weight-bearing	Stands with support, full weight not taken	Full weight taken on legs	Shifts weight from one leg to the other	Walks supported
Babbling	Silence or purposeless noise	Occasional purposeful babble	Frequent purposeful babble	Two-syllable babble	Recognizable word

Formal scales of general assessment

Bayley Scales of Infant Development (Bayley, 1965)
Age range 2 months–2½ years.

These scales were prepared very thoroughly and were carefully standardized. There are three complementary parts: the mental scale, the motor scale and the infant behaviour record. Although devised in California, USA, the scales are used extensively in the UK, where comparative standardization procedures have been carried out (Francis-Williams and Yule, 1967).

Exam. at 30 months	Date ....

Mother's Comments			
	Happy	No	Yes
	Sleeps	No	Yes
	Eats	No	Yes
Illness since last exam. (if yes specify nature of illness)	Imaginative Play	No	Yes
....		No	Yes
Change in family circumstances		No	Yes

			NEVER	STOMES	TIMES	ALWAYS
Playgroup	No	Yes				
Nursery	No	Yes				
Minder	No	Yes				
Hours worked per week (Mother)						

	Eating Mode	Knife				
		Fork				
		Spoon				
	Bowels	D				
		N				
	Bladder	D				
		N				

Reported Sentences (words)	1	2	3	4

Kick ball	Runs into ball		Poor kick	Good direct kick	
Throw ball	No throw	2 hands poor direct	2 hands good direct	1 hand	
Screws on table	10	8	6	4	

Vision both eyes	ROLLING BALLS				STYCAR 5 LETTER				
	1/2"	1/4"	3/16"	1/8"	6/26	6/24	6/12	6/9	6/6

Cover test	Squint		Doubtful	No Squint	
6 toy hearing	4 and under		5–6 with hesitation	6 immediate	

Speech – Ladybird Book	Vocab.	Less than 10 pictures	10 – 19 pictures	20 or more pictures
	Comprehension	Less than 3 actions	4–8 actions	9 or more actions
Sentences observed	Single words only	2 connected words	3 words	4 or more words
Foam board	2 or less in	3 in after mistakes	2 in immediately straight	3 in reversed immediately

PHYSICAL EXAM

(63–65)		Weight Kgms (66–68)			Height Cms. (69–71)			H.C. Cms.

Abnormality No/Yes (Specify below) ....

.... Dominant Foot | R | L

.... " Hand | R | L

.... " Eye | R | L

Appearance

Comments

Action

If tests incomplete because of child's unco-operation put tick in box		

Figure 14.2 Developmental screening examination at 30 months (Hooper, Curtis-Jenkins and Holt, 1984)

British Ability Scales (Elliott, Murray and Pearson, 1983)

Age range 2½–17½ years.

A series of 23 associated scales which cover the areas of speed of information processing, reasoning, spatial imagery, perceptual matching, short-term memory, and retrieval and application of knowledge.

The scales have been devised to lead on to recommendations for practical help for children with difficulties.

Columbia Mental Maturity Scale (Burgmeister, Blum and Lorge, 1972)

Age range 3½–10 years.

Test based on recognition of drawings different from others in each group. Reliable and useful because it is non-verbal and not strongly culturally biased.

Gesell Developmental Schedules (Gesell and Amatruda, 1969)

Age range 0–5 years.

Designed for use by paediatricians who must, however, receive appropriate training.

These scales have a clinical diagnostic orientation and, being more concerned with the diagnosis and evaluation of abnormalities than with the measurement of attainment, they are more satisfactorily applicable to handicapped children than are some of the other tests.

There is a bias towards motor items especially in the first 2 years. The results are presented in four areas: motor, adaptive, language and personal–social.

Goodenough Draw-a-Man Test (Harris, 1963)

Age range 3–15 years.

This is a simple, interesting and easily administered test, which the child usually enjoys. The child is presented with a crayon and paper and encouraged to draw a man. By showing the child what is required, the test can be entirely independent of verbal instructions. Adequate manipulative skill is required. A score is derived from an analysis of the drawing and is converted to a mental age. The ease and speed of administration make this an attractive test, but it is inadvisable to use it alone because it tests only part of the range of intellectual skills. (See also Chapter 9).

Griffiths Scales (Griffiths, 1967, 1970)

Age range 0–7 years.

There are two consecutive scales. They are designed for use by clinicians who have received appropriate training. They are attractive tests with a strong developmental emphasis and presentation of the observations in five areas.

The 'infant' scale, is widely used and well liked, but the extension scale is not so familiar and it is possibly not quite as good as some of the other tests available for this age range, with rather too many of the performance items being timed tests.

McCarthy Scales of Children's Abilities (McCarthy, 1972)

Age range 2½–8½ years.

Tests grouped in six areas: verbal, perceptual, performance, quantitative, memory, motor and general cognitive. Tends to be performance biased.

Merrill–Palmer Scale of Mental Tests (Stutsman, 1948)

Age range 18 months–6 years.

The material of this test is attractive. The test taps various abilities, but the results are not presented in subsections. Considerable reliance is placed upon speed by the inclusion of many timed items, and this makes the test less satisfactory for children with physical disabilities.

Raven's Progressive Matrices (Raven, 1939)
Age range: standard 8½ years–adult; coloured 5–11 years

These tests are very easy for a child to understand, so there is seldom any difficulty in administration or scoring. Many examiners like the matrices because of their lack of cultural bias and the fact that they do not require language for their administration and completion. The matrices test is often used in conjunction with the Mill Hill Vocabulary Scale, which indicates how well that capacity has been realized in a particular cultural environment.

Stanford–Binet Intelligence Scale (Terman and Merrill, 1961)
This is a very well-known test of general intelligence which is used extensively in the British education services. It correlates well with educational attainments. It has a verbal bias which renders it unsuitable for some children as a measure of their possible intellectual potential; for example, those with language disorders, and immigrant children for whom English is not their mother tongue. There are a wide variety of test items, some of which could be made more interesting.

Wechsler Intelligence Scales for Children (WISC) (Wechsler, 1974)
Age range 6–17 years.

The age range is extended at the younger end to 4 years by the Wechsler Preschool and Primary Scale of Intelligence (WPPSI) test which is very similar to the WISC.

The WISC has been used very widely for many years and is relied upon a great deal. The WPPSI is designed to discriminate between children aged 4–6 years. The distinctive feature of both scales is the separate examination of verbal and performance intelligence. Although this was an advance upon methods measuring general intelligence, it may perhaps have led to too great a separation of these two aspects which are, in fact, interrelated in many ways. The tests rely upon the presentation of the same task in increasingly complex forms until the child's limit is reached. This method sometimes frustrates the child and leads to blocking.

Tests of language abilities

Language assessment is one of the most difficult areas of clinical assessment because many features have to be examined, and there is considerable variation between individuals (Yule and Rutter, 1987). The features which have to be examined include the following:

ability to hear;
desire to listen;
ability to discriminate word sounds;
comprehension of increasingly complex verbal utterances;
ability to attach verbal labels to objects;
ability to form verbal concepts;
ability to link verbal concepts;
ability to formulate verbal responses;
ability to organize expressive language;
ability to articulate verbal expressions.

There are several reasons for the variations in language development which exist. Genetic influences play some part. Overall, girls show more advanced language development in their early years than boys. Environmental factors play a considerable part by influencing the pattern and frequency of opportunities to explore language, and by stimulating or inhibiting the child's desires to communicate and to express himself.

Paediatricians will be alerted to the need for further investigation when:

(a) the parents make definite complaints about some aspects of language development;
(b) a child appears not to hear or does not attempt to listen;
(c) a child by 12 months of age not responding to his name, or not understanding 'No', or not making at least one response to a clue word such as 'shoe' (e.g. 'Where's baby's shoe?');
(d) a child by 18 months of age not producing at least one or two words;
(e) a child by 2 years of age not showing any appreciation of symbolic representation (e.g. a doll, spoon, cup are not recognized for what they are);
(f) a child by 3 years of age not listening to a story, unable to carry out verbal requests, or unable to understand positional prepositions such as 'inside', 'underneath' and 'beside', and unable to use phrases of two or three words;
(g) a child of 3 years of age or more producing a flow of speech which is not related to the situation.

Hearing and auditory reception

Prior to the investigation of language impairment, it is essential to show that the child can hear and understand what is said.

Audiometry is the basis of the hearing tests.

Various sound, word and sentence descrimination tests have been developed (Templin, 1957; Sheridan, 1958; Wepman, 1958; Morgan-Barry, 1988).

Expression

Training and experience is necessary in order to make a reliable evaluation of a child's expression. Note should be made of clarity and intelligibility, content, phonology, and phrase and sentence structure.

Tests used include:

1. Mean Length of Utterance (Miller, 1981).
2. Edinburgh Articulation Test (Anthony et al., 1971).
3. Language Assessment, Remediation and Screening Procedure (Crystal, 1979; Bishop, 1984).

Short clinical procedures to identify language disorders

Drs P. Zinkin and C. Cox (1975, personal communication), in the author's department, followed the development of young children and used the items shown in Table 14.3 in their examination.

Pollak (1972) carried out a study of the development of 3-year-old children in South London which highlighted the serious language deficits of West Indian children. She used a book (*'I See a Lot of Things'*, Netherlands: L. Van Leer, 1966)

Table 14.3 Hearing, speech and language items from the developmental schedules of the 'Hounslow' study (Zinkin, 1975)

At 2 years

COMPREHENSION
Identifies:	ball, brush, cup, doll, car, spoon
Obeys:	Put the spoon in the cup
	Put the brush in the box
	Put the lid on the box

EXPRESSION
Names:	ball, brush, cup, doll, car, spoon
Spontaneous speech:	simple words, phrases

SYMBOLIZATION
Spontaneous play:	Observed
Guided play:	Give dolly a drink

At 3 years

COMPREHENSION
Identifies:	what we sit on, drink from, cut with, write with, eat with, ride in
Obeys:	Show me the biggest balloon
	Put the penny underneath the cup

EXPRESSION   Spontaneous sentences as heard

containing attractive full-page colour photographs of everyday objects. There were 25 objects altogether which the 3-year-old children were asked to identify, and they were also asked the purpose of some of them. She asked each child to recite a nursery rhyme and asked several questions about personal identity such as 'What is your name?'. Several familiar objects were given to the children, who were asked to name them and say how they were used. The children were asked to perform simple actions to show their comprehension of adverbs and to repeat three digits. Throughout the test their spontaneous speech was noted. Pollak awarded 1 point for each of 14 items which she expected the 3-year-old children to pass. The mean

Table 14.4 Pollak's items for testing the language attainment of 3-year-old children (one point is awarded for each item passed by the child)

Can name 22 out of 25 pictures
Can give purpose of 7 out of 8 objects
Recite most of one nursery rhyme
Sings a song
Knows his full name
Knows own sex
Names his mother
Names doctor
Is heard to use sentences of three or more words
Calls himself 'I'
Names 6 out of 7 objects
Correctly answers 6 out of 7 questions about everyday objects
Knows meaning of two adverbs
Can repeat three sets of three digits

score of 3-year-old children in English families was 12.04, showing that normal 3-year-old children reared in English families were able to pass most of the test items. In contrast, the 3-year-olds of West Indian families reared in London achieved a mean score of only 3.85. The 14 items are shown in Table 14.4.

Cash (1975) devised a language screening test for 3-year-old children while studying at The Wolfson Centre. His scheme was based upon Reynell's work, and is shown in Figure 14.3. Cash's test includes items pertinent to each stage of language comprehension and expression.

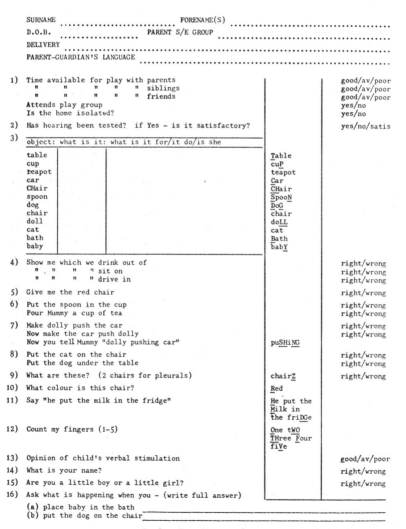

Figure 14.3 A language scale for 3-year-old children (Cash, 1975)

Bzoch–League Receptive Expressive Emergent Language Scale (Bzoch and League, 1971)

Age range 0–3 years.

There are three items of both reception and expression for each month in the first year, every 2 months in the second year and every 3 months in the third year. For example:

16–18 months

R43. Comprehends simple questions and carries out two consecutive directions with a ball or other object.

R44. Remembers and associates new words by categories (such as food, clothing, animals, etc.).

R45. From a single request identifies 2 or more familiar objects from a group of 4 or more.

E43. Begins using words rather than gestures to express wants and needs.

E44. Begins repeating words overheard in conversations.

E45. Evidences a continual but gradual increase in speaking vocabulary.

Stycar Language Test (Sheridan, 1975)

Sheridan bases her test upon four codes of communication. The principal one is the *verbal code*. The others are the *pictorial code,* the *mimed code,* both improvized and systematized forms, and the *model representative code.* The development of these codes, especially the verbal and pictorial codes, as summarized by Sheridan is shown in Table 9.14 (pages 126–127). This shows the evolution of spoken language and is concerned principally with the verbal code, but the importance of the pictorial code is shown in the child's interest in pictures and his use of drawings of people and everyday situations. The mimed code appears early when pointing is used to reinforce verbal expression (14 months), and the model representative code applies in the play situations with miniature toys.

The test consists of three overlapping procedures: the Common Objects Test (1–2 years); the Miniature Toys Test (21 months–4½ years); and the Picture Book Test (2½–7 years). Sheridan emphasizes that the Stycar Language Test is neither a screening test nor a pass/fail type of test. Rather, it is intended to provide a descriptive profile for clinical assessment and must be used by examiners with sound experienced clinical judgement.

Reynell Developmental Language Scales (Reynell, 1969)

Age range 1–7 years.

These scales were created for the assessment of the two most important central language processes – verbal comprehension and expressive language. Each scale consists of sections arranged in developmental sequence and increasing complexity. During the test a child will pass some of the early items and then reach a point beyond which he cannot pass. The score of the items passed indicates the developmental level.

The sections of the verbal comprehension scale are as follows:

1. Verbal preconcepts:
    (a) Response (e.g. change of facial expression) to familiar vocalization.

       (b) Association of particular vocalization with a particular situation (e.g. turning to door in response to 'Daddy coming').

       (c) Word pattern associated with particular object or person in a single context (e.g. 'Where's your shoe?' evokes looking at shoe only when it is on the foot).

2.   Verbal labelling of familiar objects (e.g. 'cup', 'ball', 'doll').

3.   Internalized verbal concepts (a particular word is applied to all objects and models having similar features, e.g. 'dog' applied to all dogs).

4.   Relation of two verbal concepts (e.g. put the *spoon* in the *cup*).

5.   Interpretation of question into subjective action related to the perceived object (e.g. 'Which one do we sweep the floor with?' – child has to identify the brush).

6–8. Increasing elaboration of intellectualization of language processes (e.g. 'Which one cooks the dinner?'; 'Put the penny underneath the cup'; 'Put all the pigs in the box and give me a brown horse').

9.   Recreation of situations and their solution (e.g. 'This little boy has spilt his dinner. What must he do?').

The sections of the expressive language scale are as follows:

1.   Language structure:
       (a) Vocalization.
       (b) Single-syllable sounds.
       (c) Two different sounds.
       (d) Four different sounds.
       (e) Double-syllable babble (e.g. 'mum-mum').
       (f) One definite word.
       (g) Expressive jargon (defined as patterned vocalization simulating speech).
       (h) Estimate of number of words produced.
       (i) Word combination.
       (j) Sentences of 4 or more syllables.
       (k) Words other than nouns or verbs.
       (l) Correct use of pronouns, prepositions, questions.
       (m) Correct order of words in sentence with no omission.
       (n) Use of complex sentences.

2.   Vocabulary:
       (a) Elicited with objects.
       (b) Elicited with pictures.
       (c) Elicited with words.

3.   Language content.

Illinois Test of Psycholinguistic Abilities (Kirk and Kirk, 1971)
Age range 2–10 years.

This is a lengthy and complex test which explores the communication pathways and provides information about auditory-vocal and auditory-motor functions, and the organization of both receptive and expressive language functions. It may appear to provide a more precise analysis than in fact it does; it has a cultural bias; and it may become tedious for the child, the examiner or both. Despite these criticisms, it is a sophisticated investigative tool which used by experienced psychologists in correctly selected cases yields valuable information.

British Picture Vocabulary Test (BPVT) (Dunn *et al.*, 1982)
Age range 2½–18 years.

A simple attractive test which is easily and quickly administered. It provides a useful means of exploring the extent and nature of a child's verbal understanding without his needing to use expressive language. The test is limited if the child has not experienced the items illustrated. This test seems to be used quite often by teachers.

Test for Reception of Grammar (TROG) (Bishop, 1983)
Age range 4–12 years.

The test is designed to assess understanding of grammatical contrasts in English. From 80 test items, each consisting of pictures, subjects select the one corresponding to the spoken phrase or sentence. The test reveals levels of comprehension and also specific areas of difficulty.

Symbolic Play Test (Lowe and Costello, 1988)
Age range 1–3 years.

An objective test exploring early concept formation and symbolization and providing an evaluation of pre-language skills.

Tests of reading ability (Vincent *et al.*, 1983; Vincent, 1984)

Tests of reading ability have been available for some time, but more have been devised recently and old ones have been brought up-to-date. Those in frequent use include the following:

Schonell Graded Word Reading Test (Schonell and Goodacre, 1974)
(See Chapter 11).

Standard Reading Tests (Daniels and Diack, 1971)
These consist of a standard test designed to show the level of reading competence and to expose particular difficulties, backed up by 11 diagnostic tests covering: copying of abstract figures and sentences, visual discrimination and orientation, letter recognition, aural discrimination, word recognition both verbal and pictorial, silent prose reading and comprehension, graded spelling and reading.

Neale Analysis of Reading Ability (Neale, 1989)
A recently updated well-established individual reading test.

Reading Ability Scales (NFER, 1989) *and Suffolk Reading Scale* (Hagley, 1989)
Both these scales are designed for group administration.

Tests of motor skills

Bruininks–Oseretsky Test of Motor Proficiency (Bruininks, 1978)
Age range 4–14½ years.

This test is a refinement of the original Oseretsky tests. Normative data are available. Eight areas are examined: running, speed and agility; balance; bilateral co-ordination; strength; upper limb co-ordination; response speed; visual motor control; upper limb speed and dexterity.

Test of Motor Proficiency (Gubbay, 1975)
A quick test designed for use by clinicians to detect children with motor impairment. Eight items are checked: whistle through pointed lips; skip forward 5 steps; roll ball with foot; throw, clap hands and then catch tennis ball; tie shoelace with double bow; thread 10 beads; pierce 20 pinholes; use posting box.

Test of Motor Impairment (Stott, Moyes and Henderson, 1984)
Age range 5–13 years.
   Derived from the original Oseretsky test. Five aspects of motor function are examined in the original test: control and balance (body immobile); control and co-ordination of upper limbs; control and co-ordination with body in motion; manual dexterity; tasks of simultaneous movements and precision. In the revised version, activities are divided into eight categories. The test is a useful measure of motor impairment.

Test of Minor Neurological Dysfunction (Touwen, 1979)
Age range 3–12 years.
   An unstandardized test for use by clinicians to detect children with minor (soft) signs of possible neurological dysfunction. Really a systematized clinical neurological examination for use in the examination of clumsy children.

Kinaesthetic Sensation Tests (Laszlo and Bairstow, 1986)
Age range 5–12 years.
   Two aspects are examined: kinaesthetic acuity and kinaesthetic memory.

Perceptual-Motor Abilities Test (Laszlo and Bairstow, 1986)
Age range 5–12 years
   This is a comprehensive test which seeks out functional abilities such as spatial and temporal planning and programming, balance, response speed, and kinaesthetic awareness. The findings can be used to plan a remedial programme.

Tests of visual perception

Frostig Developmental Test of Visual Perception (Frostig et al., 1964)
Age range 4–8 years.
   It has been used for many years and is available from NFER, Windsor.

Bender Visual Motor Gestalt Test (Bender, 1938)
Age range 4 years–adult.
   The Bender test has been used for many years, and in addition to information about visuo-motor competence it has been adapted to provide evaluation of development, brain injury and emotional disturbance.

References
Anthony, A., Bogle, D., Ingram, T. T. S. and McIsaac, M. W. (1971) *The Edinburgh Articulation Test*. Edinburgh: Churchill Livingstone

Bayley, N. (1965) Comparisons of mental and motor test scores for ages 1–15 months by sex, birth, order and race, geographical location and education of parents. *Child Dev.,* **36,** 379

Bellman, M. and Cash, J. (1987). *The Schedule of Growing Skills in Practice.* Windsor: NFER/Nelson

Bender, L. A. (1938) A visual motor gestalt test and its clinical use. *American Orthopsychiatric Association Research Monograph,* No. 3. New York: AOAR

Bishop, D. V. M. (1983) *T.R.O.G. Manual.* Abingdon: Thomas Leach

Bishop, D. V. M. (1984) Automated LARSP computer assisted grammatical analysis. *Br. J. Dis. Comm.,* **19,** 78–87

Bruininks, R. H. (1978) *Bruininks–Oseretsky Test of Motor Proficiency.* Circle Pines, Minnesota: American Guidance Service

Bryant, G. M., Davies, K. J. and Newcombe, R. G. (1974) The Denver Developmental Screening Test: achievement of test items in the first year of life by Denver and Cardiff infants. *Devl. Med. Child Neurol.,* **16,** 475

Burgmeister, B. B., Blum, L. H. and Lorge, I. (1972) *Columbia Mental Maturity Scale,* 3rd edn. New York: Harcourt, Brace, Jovanovich.

Bzoch, K. R. and League, R. (1971) *Assessing Language Skills in Infancy.* Gainsville, Florida: Tree of Life Press

Cash, J. (1975) A screening test of language development in three year olds. *Dissertation.* London: The Wolfson Centre/Institute of Child Health, University of London

Crystal, D. (1979) *Working with Language Assessment Remediation and Screening Procedure.* London: Edward Arnold

Daniels, J. C. and Diack, H. (1971) *The Standard Reading Tests.* London: Chatto and Windus

Dunn, L., Dunn, L., Whelton, C. and Pintilie, D. (1982) *British Picture Vocabulary Test.* Windsor: NFER/Nelson

Egan, D. F. and Brown, R. (1984) Developmental assessment: eighteen months to 4½ years. The Bus Puzzle test. *Child Care Hlth Dev.,* **10,** 381–390

Elliott, C. D., Murray, D. J. and Pearson, L. S. (1983) *British Ability Scales – Revised.* Windsor: NFER/Nelson

Francis-Williams, J. and Yule, W. (1967) The Bayley Infant Scales of Mental and Motor Development. *Devl. Med. Child Neurol.,* **9,** 391

Frankenberg, W. K. and Dodds, J. B. (1968) *The Denver Developmental Screening Test.* Denver: University of Colorado Press

Frostig, M., Maslow, P., Lefever D. W. and Whittlesey, J. R. B. (1964). The Marrainne Frostig Developmental Test of Visual Perception. *Perceptual and Motor Skills,* **19,** 463–499

Gesell, A. and Amatruda, C. S. (1969) *Developmental Diagnosis.* New York: Harper and Row

Griffiths, R. (1967) *The Abilities of Babies,* 4th edn. London: University of London Press

Griffiths, R. (1970) *The Abilities of Young Children.* Chard, Somerset: Young and Son

Gubbay, S. S. (1975) *The Clumsy Child. A Study of Developmental Apraxia and Agnosic Ataxia.* London: W. B. Saunders

Hagley, F. (1989) *Suffolk Reading Scale.* Windsor: NFER/Nelson

Harris, D. B. (1963) *Children's Drawings as Measures of Intellectual Maturity.* New York: Harcourt, Brace and World

Holt, K. S. and Reynell, J. (1967) *Observation of Chidren.* London: National Association for Mental Health

Hooper, P., Curtis-Jenkins, G. and Holt, K. S. (1984) *Developmental Surveillance in Pre-school Children.* Report to DHSS, London

Kirk, S. A. and Kirk, W. D. (1971) *Psycholinguistic Learning Difficulties. Diagnosis and Remediation.* Chicago: University of Illinois Press

Laszlo, J. I. and Bairstow, P. (1986) *Perceptual Motor Behaviour.* London: Holt, Rinehart and Winston

Lingam, S. (1987) *Its Your Life – A Parent Held Child Health Record.* Singapore: Eltan Publishing

Lowe, M. and Costello, A. (1988) *Symbolic Play Test,* 2nd edn. Windsor: NFER

McCarthy, D. A. (1972) *Manual for the McCarthy Scales of Children's Abilities.* New York: Psychological Corporation

Miller, J. F. (1981) *Assessing Language Production in Children: Experimental Procedures.* Baltimore: University Park Press

Morgan-Barry, R. (1988) *Auditory Discrimination and Attention Test.* Windsor: NRER/Nelson

Neale, M. D. (1989) *Neale Analysis of Reading Ability.* Windsor: NFER/Nelson

NFER (1989) *Reading Ability Series.* Windsor: NFER/Nelson

Pollak, M. (1972) *Today's Three Year Olds in London.* London: Heinemann

Raven, J. C. (1939) The R.E.C.I. series of perceptual tests: an experimental survey. *Br. J. Med. Psychol.,* **18,** 16

Reynell, J. (1969) *Reynell Developmental Language Scales.* Windsor: NFER

Schonell, F. J. and Goodacre, E. (1974) *The Psychology and Teaching of Reading,* 5th edn. Edinburgh: Oliver and Boyd

Sheridan, M. D. (1958) *Manual of the Stycar Hearing Test.* Windsor: NFER

Sheridan, M. D. (1975) The Stycar language test. *Devl. Med. Child Neurol.,* **17,** 164

Starte, G. D. (1972) 'Child's play' or paediatric developmental assessment in general practice. *Practitioner,* **209,** 84

Stott, D. H., Moyes, F. A. and Henderson, S. E. (1984) *A Test of Motor Impairment.* Guelph, Ontario: Brook Educational Publishing

Stutsman, R. (1948) *Mental Measurement of Pre-School Children.* New York: Harcourt, Brace and World

Templin, M. (1957) *Certain Language Skills in Children.* Minneapolis, USA: University of Minnesota Press

Terman, L. M. and Merrill, M. A. (1961) *Stanford Binet Intelligence Scale.* 3rd rev. form L.M. London: Harrap

Touwen, B. C. L. (1979) Examination of the child with minor neurological dysfunction. *Clinics Dev. Med. 71.* London: Heinemann

Uzgiris, I. C. and Hunt, J. McV. (1975) *Assessment in Infancy: Ordinal Scales of Psychological Development.* Urbana, USA: University of Illinois Press

Vincent, D. (1984) *Reading Tests in the Classroom.* Windsor: NFER/Nelson

Vincent, D., Powney, J., Green, L. and Francis, J. (1983) *A Review of Reading Tests.* Windsor: NFER/Nelson

Wechsler, D. (1974) *Manual for the Wechsler Intelligence Scale for Children – revised.* New York: Psychological Corporation

Wepman, J. P. (1958) *Auditory Discrimination Test.* Chicago: Language Research Associates

Yule, W. and Rutter, M. (1987) *Language Development and Disorders. Clinics Dev. Med. 101/102.* Oxford: Blackwell Scientific Publications

Zinkin P. (1975) A study of the allocation of resources in the detection of children under 3 years with developmental delay. Descriptions and preliminary results. In *The Early Identification of Educationally 'At Risk' Children* (eds Wedell, K. and Raybould, E. C.). Occasional Publications No. 6, Birmingham: School of Education

Index